T0000439

WALKING PHILADELPHIA

30 Tours of Art, Architecture, History, and Little-Known Gems

Second Edition

Natalie Pompilio and Tricia Pompilio

 WILDERNESS PRESS ... *on the trail since 1967*

Walking Philadelphia: 30 Tours of Art, Architecture, History, and Little-Known Gems
Copyright © 2017 and 2022 by Natalie Pompilio and Tricia Pompilio
Second edition, first printing

Distributed by Publishers Group West
Manufactured in the United States of America

Cover design: Scott McGrew
Cover photo: © Sean Pavone/Shutterstock, Eugenio Marongiu/Shutterstock, and
  Shchus/Shutterstock (Independence Hall)
Interior design: Lora Westberg; typesetting: Annie Long
Interior photos: Tricia Pompilio; photo on p. 147 by Scott Biales/Shutterstock
Cartography: Steve Jones; map data: OpenStreetMap
Project and copy editor: Holly Cross
Proofreader: Emily Beaumont
Indexer: Potomac Indexing, LLC

Library of Congress Cataloging-in-Publication Data

Names: Pompilio, Natalie, author. | Pompilio, Tricia, 1975- author.
Title: Walking Philadelphia : 30 tours of art, architecture, history, and little-known gems /
  Natalie Pompilio and Tricia Pompilio
Other titles: Walking Philadelphia, thirty tours of art, architecture, history, and
  little-known gems
Description: Second edition. | Birmingham, AL : Wilderness Press, [2022] | Includes index.
Identifiers: LCCN 2022024573 (print) | LCCN 2022024574 (ebook) |
  ISBN 9781643590899 (paperback) | ISBN 9781643590905 (ebook)
Subjects: LCSH: Philadelphia (Pa.)—Tours. | Philadelphia (Pa.)—Guidebooks. |
  Walking—Pennsylvania—Philadelphia—Guidebooks. | Historic buildings—
  Pennsylvania—Philadelphia—Guidebooks. | Historic buildings—Pennsylvania—
  Philadelphia—Guidebooks. | Historic sites—Pennsylvania—Philadelphia—Guidebooks.
Classification: LCC F158.18 .P66 2022 (print) | LCC F158.18 (ebook) | DDC 917.48/1104—dc23
LC record available at https://lccn.loc.gov/2022024573
LC ebook record available at https://lccn.loc.gov/2022024574

Published by: **WILDERNESS PRESS**
              An imprint of AdventureKEEN
              2204 First Ave. S., Suite 102
              Birmingham, AL 35233
              800-678-7006, fax 877-374-9016

Visit wildernesspress.com for a complete list of our books and for ordering information. Contact
us at our website, at facebook.com/wildernesspress1967, or at twitter.com/wilderness1967 with
questions or comments. To find out more about who we are and what we're doing, visit
blog.wildernesspress.com.

SAFETY NOTICE: Although Wilderness Press and the authors have made every attempt to ensure
that the information in this book is accurate at press time, they are not responsible for any loss,
damage, injury, or inconvenience that may occur to anyone while using this book. You are responsible for your own safety and health while following the walking trips described here.

Dedication

For Mom, Patricia Pompilio, January 24, 1944–July 18, 2014

When next we meet, we'll walk together.

Acknowledgments

From Natalie: One advantage of writing about Philadelphia is the wealth of information easily found online and in the library. Writing this guide would have been much less enjoyable if I hadn't had Hidden City Philadelphia, Naked Philly, and the Association of Public Art. *The Philadelphia Inquirer* and *The Philadelphia Daily News,* both found at inquirer.com, were also essential. I found some lovely snark published in *Philadelphia* magazine. The Free Library of Philadelphia was a great resource/makeshift office. Please see the bibliography at the end for further reading. I apologize if I forgot anyone.

Thanks to everyone at AdventureKEEN—Holly Cross, Steve Jones, Annie Long, and Emily Beaumont   for editorial, production, and marketing.

Thanks to Dante Zappala, Christy Speer LeJeune, and Fon Wang for sharing their local expertise. Ellen McCusker, you're the proofreader and friend I've always dreamed of. Cara Schneider Bongiorno, let's have another nerdy history lunch soon.

My father, Lou Pompilio, promised to buy multiple copies of the book, but he did so when he thought photos of him were included. Look, Dad! I got your name in! I'm thrilled that my sister, Tricia Pompilio, could use this outlet for her fabulous photos. I hope this leads to endless opportunities. I had the support of Team Barnett/Fletcher, Katie's kettlebell class, and too many others to list. Rocky and Spike, you were faithful companions/obstructions throughout the writing process. Lisa Wathen read the finished tours and called them brilliant when they weren't.

A big shout-out to my faves: Fiona, Luna, and Poppy Savarese and Will, Maddie, and Nora Paxson. It's hard to be stressed when talking about Noisette and the No Nut Shop, playing Mr. Bowl, or making up another story about the Chewys. What would life be without Popco, Ratface's diary, and "Well, that didn't go as planned?"

Finally, I want to thank my husband, Jordan Barnett. During the mad push to finish, he made maps, made dinner, and made me laugh. Jordo, our relationship's truly special.

From Tricia: First, thank you to my talented older sister, Natalie, for making this happen. Although you were less than thrilled at my arrival 40+ years ago, you have never wavered in your support. Thank you to Rochelle Litman, my friend and neighbor. You listened patiently when I was overwhelmed, drove me around the city for hours, and acted as a constant cheerleader as I began my new career.

My kids: Fi, Lu, and Poppy. You inspire me every day. I love you more than all the stars in the sky. And thank you to my husband, Vince. Your unwavering support, love, and patience are astounding. You never complain when I disappear into my office for hours, run off on weekends for sessions, or throw my heavy camera bag on your back. I'll back you up always.

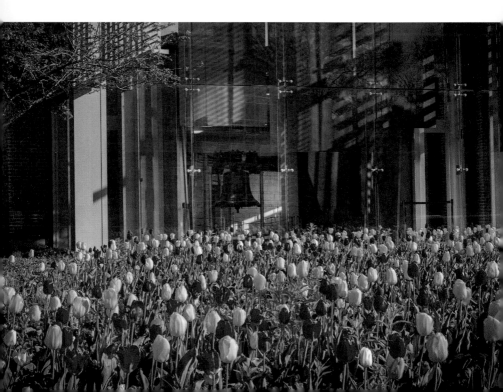

Author's Note

There are a lot of great things about living in Philadelphia. Being able to walk almost everywhere I need to go is one of them. The gym, the post office, the doctor and dentist, the grocery store, the open-air market, the pharmacy, my sister's house, my nieces' school, and more restaurants and bars than I can quickly count—none of those places is more than 1 mile from my home.

This city has hosted some of my life's biggest milestones. I thought I knew a lot about it, too, having worked here as a professional journalist and lived here as a non-professional nosy person since November 2002. I was so wrong.

Researching different neighborhoods and buildings, and the people behind them, I often found myself falling down the rabbit hole, digging deeper and deeper because it was all so interesting and new. More than once, I'd emerge from reading an original historic-designation nomination form or news clipping from the 1920s to find I'd spent more than an hour on a single stop on a single tour. I couldn't stop myself: I love tidbits and odd facts, and I'd get so excited by each one.

I was also constantly distracted because I kept thinking how tour 31 "Natalie Pompilio"—might read. One of the tours will take you within a block of my home. Another passes the hotel where my husband and I married. A third brings you to my nieces' school, and a fourth passes in front of my sister's house. I should probably include her address in case you need a bathroom.

I tried to write a walking guide that I would like to read, one that's not only fun and funny but also educational with a lot of "Wow, I didn't know that" moments. I like to imagine readers stopping in their tracks, in the middle of Rittenhouse Square or in Fishtown, and calling a friend to say, "I have to tell you about the cool thing I just read."

This book is not the definitive Philadelphia walking guide. It's a good one, yes, and a great introduction to the city. But to be definitive, it would need to include more of the city's famed neighborhoods. I started plotting my tours at the city's center and never reached the edges. Perhaps in a third edition? Until then, enjoy.

—Natalie

Table of Contents

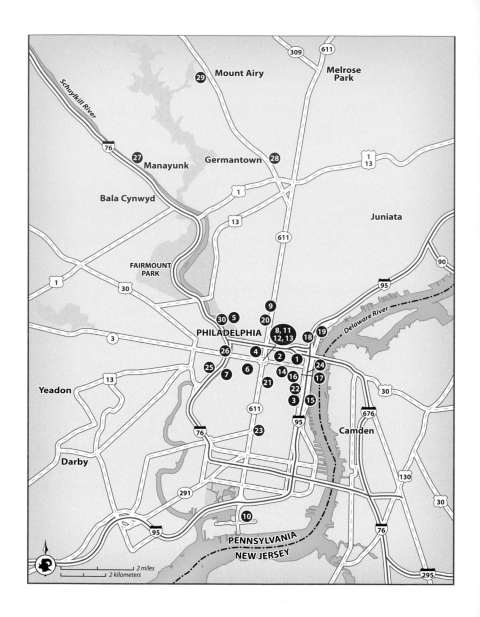

Introduction

A lot has changed in the five years since *Walking Philadelphia: 30 Walking Tours Exploring Art, Architecture, History, and Little-Known Gems* was published. That's the thing about dynamic cities like Philadelphia: Change is constant.

The global pandemic, a presidential election, and a growing social justice movement have also altered the city and its institutions. Christ Church can no longer say it has hosted an on-site Sunday service every weekend for more than 300 years. Thousands of people received COVID-19 vaccinations at the Theatre of the Living Arts and the Pennsylvania Convention Center. A statue and a mural of a controversial mayor are no longer on public display.

To update this guide, I rewalked each tour, removing places that no longer existed and changing routes to give walkers more sites to see. In the first edition, I highlighted stores and restaurants. This revised version removes most of these, giving me more room to tell stories.

In this updated version, you'll learn about a bronze bust of Benjamin Franklin made from 1,000 keys and 1.8 million pennies; America's first ransom note; and the *meschianza*, the over-the-top party that may have helped Washington's Army win the Revolutionary War. You'll explore the city's new Fashion District, stroll America's oldest residential street, and take an extended look at Girard College.

For years, many have viewed Philadelphia as New York's little sister. But consider this: The travel experts from *Travel+Leisure, Conde Nast Traveler, Fodor's,* and *Frommer's* all named Philadelphia a "must-visit destination" in 2021, noting the city's diverse neighborhoods, abundance of public art, and local restaurants that have garnered international praise.

But if you can't find time to visit until 2023 or 2024, even 2030, don't worry. Philadelphia will be here waiting—with even more to see and do.

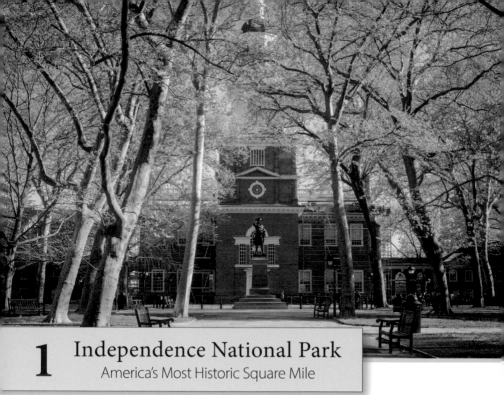

1 Independence National Park
America's Most Historic Square Mile

Above: Independence Hall is where the Declaration of Independence was signed and the US Constitution was ratified.

BOUNDARIES: Chestnut St., Race St., N. Sixth St., Front St.
DISTANCE: 1.3 miles
DIFFICULTY: Easy
PARKING: There are multiple pay lots in the area.
PUBLIC TRANSIT: The subway has a stop at Fifth and Market Sts.

Philadelphia is where the Declaration of Independence and the US Constitution were signed and ratified, where Benjamin Franklin operated a printing press and ran the local post office while experimenting with electricity, and where George Washington lived and worked during his presidency. The city is proud of its role in the shaping of America.

Walk Description

Begin at the **❶ Free Quaker Meeting House** at the corner of Arch and Fifth Streets. Philadelphia founder William Penn, who lent his family name to the Commonwealth of Pennsylvania, was a Quaker. Quakers, also called Friends, are pacifists who believe in simple lives of service. Persecuted in England, Quakers were welcomed to Philadelphia.

Free Quakers are Quakers who took up arms in the Revolutionary War and were then asked to leave their congregations, thus making them "free." They built this Georgian brick worship hall in 1783.

Look across Arch Street. The **❷ National Constitution Center** is the only museum dedicated to the US Constitution. Its live theatrical performance, *Freedom Rising,* presents US history and the country's development since the Constitution's 1787 ratification. Many exhibits are interactive. Guests can vote on Supreme Court cases or swear the presidential oath of office. The main exhibition ends in Signers' Hall, which has 42 life-size statues of the Constitution's signatories. While towering in thought, these men were short in life.

Walk east on Arch Street, crossing N. Fifth Street. **❸ Christ Church Burial Ground** is the resting place of prominent Colonial leaders, including five Declaration of Independence signatories and the founders of the United States Navy. Benjamin Franklin's grave is near the fence. Visitors throw pennies onto Franklin's flat stone, a nod to the proverb he made famous: "A penny saved is a penny earned." About 75,000 coins are tossed each year.

Look across Arch Street. The US Mint stands where the Female Anti-Slavery Society had its headquarters. Cofounded by Lucretia Mott in 1833, the organization's constitution stated, "We deem it our duty as professing Christians to manifest our abhorrence of the flagrant injustice and deep sin of slavery by united and vigorous exertions." The society disbanded in 1870 after the 15th amendment granted African American men the right to vote.

Continue east, crossing N. Fourth Street. The Arch Street Meeting House property has been actively used by Quakers since 1682. A historic marker acknowledges that it hosted the 1979 meeting of LGBTQ activists that planned the National March on Washington for Lesbian and Gay Rights. Quakers embraced the LGBTQ community, considered "toxic" at the time.

In front is a water basin installed by the Philadelphia Fountain Society in 1867 at the request of "a lady." The city once had more than 100 such fountains. About 12 remain. In the early 1870s, almost every horse in the country was infected by equine influenza, and Philadelphia was particularly hard hit because it had "one of the most extensive horse-drawn street railway systems in the nation . . . heavily reliant upon horse labor for everything from intra-urban transport of both people and goods to powering machines on construction sites," author Jeffrey Michael Flanigan writes in *On the Backs of Horses: The Great Epizootic of 1872*. An October 1872 *Philadelphia Inquirer* article said that in 15 minutes, its reporters had counted four animals "that all had the greenish colored discharge from the nostrils which indicates a development of the complaint into a somewhat serious stage." As many as 10% of the city's 50,000 horses died.

Cross Arch Street, continuing east. Sculptor James Peniston's *Keys to Community* is a 1-ton bronze bust of Benjamin Franklin made with 1,000 keys and 1.8 million pennies ($18,000) collected by local schoolchildren. It marks the entrance to Girard Fountain Park and the *History of the Philadelphia Fire Department* mural.

Continue on Arch Street, passing the former Klosfit Petticoat Factory (309–313 Arch St.). Built in 1875, it became the Hoop Skirt Factory Condos in the 1980s.

Cross N. Third Street. At the ❹ **Betsy Ross House,** a costumed Betsy reenactor works in the upholstery shop and recounts the adventures of the entrepreneur who made the nation's first flag. Nicknamed the Little Rebel, Ross also produced munitions here. Questions about the veracity of the flag claim were quashed in 2014 when curators at George Washington's Mount Vernon estate found a receipt showing Ross's shop made beddings for Washington's home, thus linking the two. Washington reportedly asked Ross to create a flag with six-pointed stars. Instead, she folded a piece of paper and, in one snip, created the five-pointed star used today.

At N. Second St., turn left. At ❺ **Elfreth's Alley,** the country's oldest continuously inhabited residential block, turn right. The 32 buildings on this narrow cobblestone street, constructed between 1720 and 1830, housed tradespeople, including furniture builders, glassblowers, and smiths. The museum here is "one of the few landmarks dedicated to the every day American," the tourism board notes. Residents open their homes to the public twice a year.

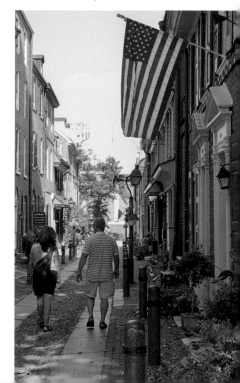

Elfreth's Alley is the oldest continuously inhabited street in the country.

Before the end of the alley, detour onto Bladen's Court on the left, which dead-ends at a small courtyard where the neighborhood's "privies" once stood.

At the end of Elfreth's Alley, turn right at N. Front Street, walking along the barrier separating I-95 traffic from downtown. At Arch Street, turn right. Pass Smythe Stores Condominiums (101–111 Arch St.) and the National (121 N. Second St.), two former industrial buildings converted to residences.

At N. Second Street, turn left, walking south. Pass Arden Theatre Company (40 N. Second St.) to reach ❻ **Christ Church**. Once called "the nation's church," it was founded in 1695, with notable early worshippers including George Washington. Until the COVID-19 shutdown of 2020, church leaders boasted that there had been a Sunday service here every weekend for more than 300 years. The 1938 children's book *Ben and Me* tells the story of Amos, a church mouse who contributed to Ben Franklin's career. Visitors still ask about the prayer book Amos allegedly nibbled.

Continue south, crossing Market Street. Stop at Chestnut Street. Ahead is the U.S. Custom House (200 Chestnut St.), the country's oldest federal agency. Many call it the *Ghostbusters* building because it resembles the Central Park West structure featured in that film.

Turn right on Chestnut Street. The Museum of the American Revolution (101 S. Third St.) sits across from Alexander Hamilton's First Bank of the United States (120 S. Third St.). Hamilton's ghost allegedly haunts the bank. After a 1902 renovation, a priest blessed the building in the hope of dispelling the spirit. Some say Hamilton's ghost is here because of guilt over the tremendous debt he'd accumulated before death that became his survivors' problem.

Continue west. Across Chestnut Street is an entrance to the ❼ **Benjamin Franklin Museum and Franklin Court**, built on the site of Franklin's home. Franklin, founder of the US Postal Service, was appointed the first Postmaster General in 1775. Cards and letters mailed here are still hand-stamped with the B. Free Franklin seal.

Continue on Chestnut Street to ❽ **Carpenters' Hall,** which in 1771 hosted the First Continental Congress, aka "the one that didn't get anything done." (The Declaration of Independence was adopted during the Second Continental Congress in 1772.) Look at the tourism placard, which shows men talking as a cat enters from the bottom right-hand corner. The First Continental Cat?

Also here is the New Hall Military Museum, a reconstruction of the first Secretary of War's office. Its exhibits trace the founding of the different branches of the Armed Forces.

Continue west. The ❾ **Second Bank of the United States,** one of the country's first Greek Revival buildings, houses a free portrait gallery.

Continue on Chestnut Street, passing Signers Garden, to ❿ **Independence Hall,** where both the Declaration of Independence and the US Constitution were signed. Its bell tower holds the

Centennial bell, made to celebrate the nation's 100th birthday. It weighs 13,000 pounds—or 1,000 pounds for each original colony—and contains metal from Revolutionary and Civil War cannons. Portraits of France's King Louis XVI and Marie Antoinette hang inside the hall, gifts from the monarchs after the Revolutionary War. The pair knew Ben Franklin, who was in France as a diplomat during most of the war. Historian Geri Walton said the 71-year-old Franklin was very popular with French women because "he was a ladies' man with a big libido."

Today, the hall is a centerpiece of the city's July Fourth celebrations. After the U.S. Supreme Court's 2015 ruling for marriage equality, lead plaintiff James Obergefell addressed a crowd here. That same year, Pope Francis spoke about immigration on its steps.

At S. Sixth Street, turn right. **11 Liberty Bell Center** is at the corner. The bell was cast in London

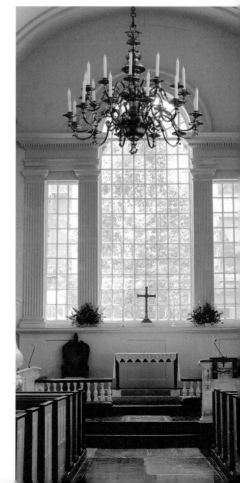

and took its place atop the Pennsylvania State House—now Independence Hall—in 1753. During the Revolutionary War, Philadelphians feared the British would melt the city's bells to make munitions, so a group took that bell and 10 others to Allentown, hiding them under a church's floorboards. The bells were returned to the city in 1778. It's unclear when the Liberty Bell began to crack—some say the fissure began soon after it arrived in Philadelphia—but it is known that the crack worsened in February 1846, when it was rung to celebrate Washington's 114th birthday.

Continue to Market Street. The brick mansion that stood on this corner housed George Washington for seven years and John Adams for three before the capital moved to Washington, D.C. In 2007, an excavation uncovered the foundations of slave quarters. Exhibits in the open-air President's House pavilion feature these enslaved workers. The walk ends here, across from Independence Visitor Center.

Christ Church is sometimes called the nation's church.

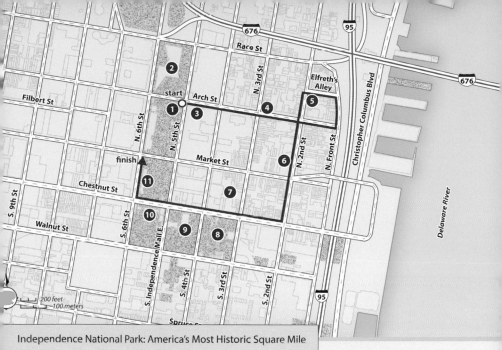

Independence National Park: America's Most Historic Square Mile

Points of Interest

1. **Free Quaker Meeting House** 500 Arch St., 215-629-5801, nps.gov/inde
2. **National Constitution Center** 525 Arch St., 215-409-6600, constitutioncenter.org
3. **Christ Church Burial Ground** Arch and N. Fifth Sts.
4. **Betsy Ross House** 239 Arch St., 215-629-4026, historicphiladelphia.org/betsy-ross-house/what-to-see
5. **Elfreth's Alley** N. Second St. between Race and Arch Sts.
6. **Christ Church** 20 N. American St., 215-922-1695, christchurchphila.org
7. **Benjamin Franklin Museum and Franklin Court** 317 Chestnut St., 267-514-1522, nps.gov/inde
8. **Carpenters' Hall** 320 Chestnut St., 215-925-0167, carpentershall.org
9. **Second Bank of the United States** 420 Chestnut St.
10. **Independence Hall** 520 Chestnut St., 215-965-2305, nps.gov/inde
11. **Liberty Bell Center** S. Sixth and Market Sts., 215-965-2305, nps.gov/inde

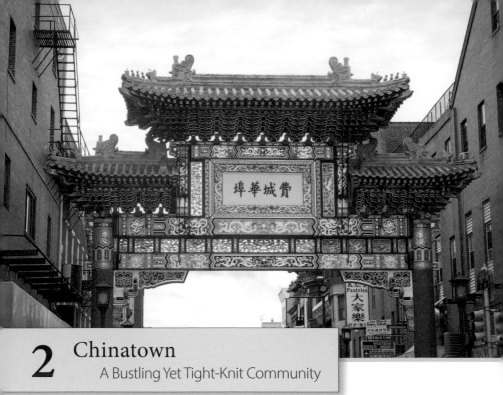

2 Chinatown
A Bustling Yet Tight-Knit Community

Above: Chinatown's Friendship Gate was a gift from Philadelphia's sister city of Tianjin, China.

BOUNDARIES: Vine St., Arch St., N. 11th St., N. Eighth St.
DISTANCE: 1.1 miles
DIFFICULTY: Easy
PARKING: Street parking in this area is difficult. There are pay lots nearby.
PUBLIC TRANSIT: SEPTA bus lines that stop in Chinatown include the 23, 47, 48, and 61. The SEPTA Chinatown subway stop is also nearby.

Philadelphia's Chinatown was established in the 1870s when Chinese immigrants from the West Coast moved east to escape growing anti-Chinese sentiment and violence, a migration known as The Driving Out.

Today, this is the East Coast's third-largest Chinatown. Residents have battled multiple government attempts to upend it and have largely avoided the gentrification that has occurred in the Chinatowns of New York and Boston. About 3,000 people live here, the vast majority of Asian descent, including those of Korean, Vietnamese, Burmese, Japanese, and Malaysian origin. It's a tight-knit group. They say if you bring any 20 neighbors together, 5 of them will be related—or at least as close as family.

Walk Description

Start at **❶ Chinatown Friendship Gate,** which rises four stories and then curves over North 10th Street at Arch Street. This 40-foot-tall authentic Chinese gate, dedicated in 1984, was a gift from Philadelphia's sister city, Tianjin, China. The multicolored carvings include dragons and a phoenix. The four Chinese characters spell "Philadelphia Chinatown." In 2008, artisans from Tianjin spent four months restoring the gate. They used traditional Chinese methods, including fresh pigs' blood as paint primer.

Walk north on North 10th Street. The sidewalk panels bear the Chinese symbol for prosperity in red outlined in black. These can also be seen on the low wall separating Chinatown from the Vine Street Expressway.

The building at 125 N. 10th Street, constructed in 1831, housed the Chinatown YMCA. Its owner, Chinese-born T. T. Chang, was known as "the mayor of Chinatown" for his work improving residents' lives. Inscribed to the door's right is "1970" and the corresponding Chinese calendar year of "4668." That year the building exterior was given Mandarin Palace accents by C. C. Yang, an influential 20th-century architect. Changes included a jade colored glazed tile awning on the first floor, red balconies, a gabled roof, and red entry doors with lion's head door knockers.

Turn left onto Cherry Street **❷ Fo Shou Buddhist Temple** features red columns of coiling dragons and flying eaves. Open daily, the first floor features three golden Buddhas, while the top has an ancestral shrine, a nod to the Chinese practice of combining ancestor worship and Confucianism. (Other businesses have similar altars.)

Return to North 10th Street. For a beverage, stop at **❸ Tea Dó,** a contemporary teahouse offering bubble teas and snacks. Across the street, the Philadelphia Fire Department's Engine 20/ Ladder 23 is called the House of Dragons. Why would a flame-spewing animal be the symbol of an organization dedicated to fighting fires? Because in Chinese mythology, dragons control water, including rain and the flow of water from a hose. Dragons bring life-giving water to the people who honor and respect them while punishing enemies with hurricanes and floods.

Continue north, turning left on Race Street. Note the Chinese characters spelling out the road's name. **❹ David's Mai Lai Wah** is one of the neighborhood's original late-night dining spots, open most days until 4 a.m. The owner has admitted he sometimes closes the shop and goes to South Philly for a cheesesteak.

Continue on Race Street. The building at 1010–1014 formerly housed the Heywood Chair Factory, which began operation in 1892. The factory, known for its high-quality products, is now condominiums and another example of how buildings from the city's manufacturing days have been repurposed.

❺ **Dim Sum Garden** specializes in *xiao long bao,* or soup dumplings from Shanghai. Owner Shizhou Da says she is descended from the first chef to make soup dumplings and hers is an original recipe passed down through five generations. Da worked in restaurants in China for 30 years and has made dumplings here since 2013. Fans recommend the Shanghai crab or pork soup dumplings.

Turn right on North 11th Street. Pass ❻ **Yakitori Boy,** an *izakaya* (a Japanese pub serving small plates and alcohol) and upscale karaoke lounge. Across the road, Chinatown Beer Garden (210 N. 11th St.) has a menu offering more than 25 Asian-made brews, including Vietnam's Bia Saigan, Korea's Kloud, Thailand's Singha, and Japan's Otaru.

At Spring Street, make a right for a quick detour to see the happy, hand-holding children featured in *A Thousand Children Playing* on the east wall of the Chinatown Learning Center (1034–36 Spring St.), aka the Bird Building. Hidden City Philadelphia details the building's commercial history; in 1917, for example, it housed the Deluxe Brush Company, the Fletching Printing Company, and the Walter F. Ware Company, a medical supply firm known for the Mizpah, a continuous suction breast pump considered a technological marvel.

Return to North 11th Street. Walk north to Winter Street and turn right. The 6th Police District, at North 11th and Winter Streets, has a mural dedicated to Officer Daniel Faulkner, who was killed on duty in 1981.

At North 10th Street, turn right. The bronze sidewalk medallions represent the animals of the Chinese zodiac. The ❼ **Chinese Christian Church** sits at the corner with Mitzi Mackenzie Place/ Spring Street. Maribelle "Mitzi" Mackenzie, who died in 2009 at age 88, was an American Baptist Home missionary. In 1941, she founded a center to aid Chinese immigrants and is credited with helping thousands of immigrants find their way. This church grew from that ministry.

Continue, passing On Lok House (219 N. 10th St.), which has provided low-income housing and social services for seniors since 1985. It exists in part thanks to Rev. Dr. Yam Tong Ho, whose personal papers, housed at the Historical Society of Pennsylvania, show "the challenges he faced in trying to find affordable housing for elderly couples living in attics without heat in the winter or air-conditioning during Philadelphia's sweltering summers and for old men with no relatives in the country trying to get by in small rooms with no readily accessible cooking or bathroom facilities," according to hsp.org.

At Race Street, turn left. In 1870, Chinese immigrant Lee Fong opened a laundry at 913 Race Street. It was the neighborhood's first Chinese-owned business. A few years later, one of Fong's relatives opened a restaurant on the building's second floor. That was followed by a few Chinese groceries and so on and so on. . . .

At North Ninth Street, turn right. At Arch Street, turn left where four dragons twist in the air. These 1,500-pound bronze beasts were installed in 2009. The Pennsylvania Department of Transportation building (801 Arch St.) was a brothel in the mid-1800s. According to *A Guide to the Stranger or Pocket Companion for the Fancy,* a collection of reviews of city brothels published in 1849, this business "had a reputation of being A No. 1 in terms of cleanliness, quietness and privacy."

Across the road is Francis House of Peace (810 Arch St.), opened in 2015 and named for Pope Francis. The building has 94 affordable housing units and offers social services in English, Mandarin, and Cantonese. The words "None of us are home until all of us are home," written in English and Chinese, is local nonprofit Project HOME's motto.

At North Eighth Street, turn left. **8** *How We Fish* (125 N. Eighth St.) honors the history of work in Philadelphia. The placement is significant: this building was originally constructed for children of workers of the International Ladies Garment Workers Union and the Amalgamated Men's Clothing Union. The garment industry is highlighted in the mural, as is denim, considered the fabric of the working class. The title comes from the proverb, "Give a man a fish, he eats for a day. Teach a man to fish, he eats for a lifetime." The eye-catching work spans 3,156 feet and includes 400 square feet of glass mosaics and the words "Work unites us."

Continue north. The Philadelphia Police Administration Building (750 Race St.) is called "the Roundhouse" and has been a polarizing structure since its completion in 1963. As public radio station WHYY asked in 2016, "Is the Roundhouse a cruel, handcuff-shaped structure with bad baggage, or is it a proud example of Philadelphia modernism, optimistic and sculptural?"

Cross Race Street. Metro Club condominiums (201 N. Eighth St.) was Metropolitan Hospital before the medical center closed in 1992. It was reborn as condominiums in 2004 after a $30 million investment.

At Vine Street, turn left. Cross North Ninth Street, passing **9** Sang Kee Peking Duck House. In 2017, the restaurant's founders, Michael and Diane Chow were the first Chinese-Americans to win the Philadelphia Welcoming Center's "Realizing the American Dream" award.

Continue west. **10** *History of Chinatown,* at North 10th and Winter Streets, was commissioned in 1995 for Chinatown's 125th anniversary. Its placement is defiant, a staking of territory after city officials divided the neighborhood with the Vine Street Expressway. At top is a laundry worker—the first Chinese settler here in the 1800s opened a laundry business at 913 Race Street.

The water drops flow to show families, a highway, and protesters carrying signs that say HOMES NOT HIGHWAYS in front of bulldozers.

Cross Vine Street Expressway's eastbound lanes to reach 10th Street Plaza, where two 7-ton Chinese foo dogs stand guard. When the plaza was dedicated in 2011, a Buddhist monk dabbed red ink on the lions' faces to awaken them as neighborhood protectors. The female rests her paw on a cub. The male's paw is on a globe. An Asian-style pergola provides shady seating.

The statue of Lin Zebu honors the scholar known for his opposition to opium smuggling. In 1838, he supervised the destruction of 20,000 chests of opium marked for Britain, sparking the first opium war between Britain and China.

The mural covering the plaza's ground, including play spaces with bilingual prompts and a neighborhood map, was completed in 2021.

Cross the Vine Street Expressway's westbound lanes. At left is the 20-story ⑪ **Crane Chinatown,** a community and recreation space opened in 2019. In a WHYY op-ed, community planner Sarah Yeung said the building provided a gymnasium for schoolchildren who formerly played in a parking lot, a large practice space for elders who once did tai chi in a cramped room, and a rooftop event space where locals could host events with citywide views. "Celebrate with us," Yeung wrote, "because for the first time, our community will have a place to call its own."

Turn right. The walk ends at ⑫ **Holy Redeemer Chinese Catholic Church.** The first Western Hemisphere church built specifically for Chinese Catholics, it opened in 1941. In 1939, Bishop Nankin, China's vicar, Paul Yu Pin, visited Philadelphia and asked to meet with its few Chinese-Catholic residents. The Philadelphia Archdiocese then focused recruitment efforts on the community, with its vice chancellor immediately gathering 15 Chinese immigrants and teaching them the sign of the cross. According to the church's website, nine Chinatown residents were baptized in October of 1939. A few months later, more than 50 others were ready for confirmation. Today, about 200 people attend Masses conducted in English, Cantonese, and Mandarin. The church school has about 250 students.

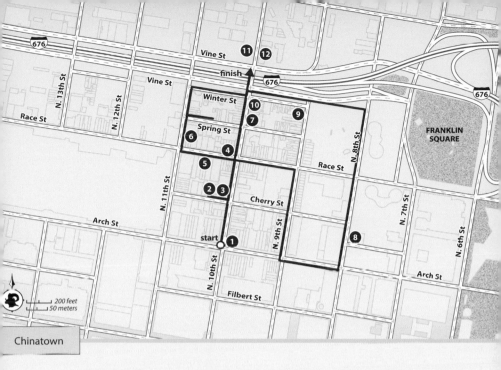

Chinatown

Points of Interest

1. **Chinatown Friendship Gate** N. 10th and Arch Sts. For more information, contact the Chinatown Development Corporation 215-922-2156, chinatown-pcdc.org.

2. **Fo Shou Buddhist Temple** 1015 Cherry St., 215-928-0592

3. **Tea Dó** 132 N. 10th St., 215-925-8889, tea-do.com

4. **David's Mai Lai Wah** 1001 Race St., 215-627-2610

5. **Dim Sum Garden** 1020 Race St., 215-873-0258, dimsumgardenphilly.com

6. **Yakitori Boy** 211 N. 11th St., 215-923-8088, yakitoriboy.com

7. **Chinese Christian Church** 225 N. 10th St., 215-627-2360, cccnc.org

8. *How We Fish* 125 N. Eighth St., Mural Arts Philadelphia, 215-685-0750, muralarts.org

9. **Sang Kee Peking Duck House** 238 N. Ninth St., 215-925-7532, sangkeechinatown.com

10. *History of Chinatown* N. 10th and Winter Sts., Mural Arts Philadelphia, 215-685-0750, muralarts.org

11. **Crane Chinatown** 1001 Vine St., 215-922-1156, facebook.com/CraneCommunityCenter

12. **Holy Redeemer Chinese Catholic Church** 915 Vine St., 215-922-0999, holyredeemer.cc

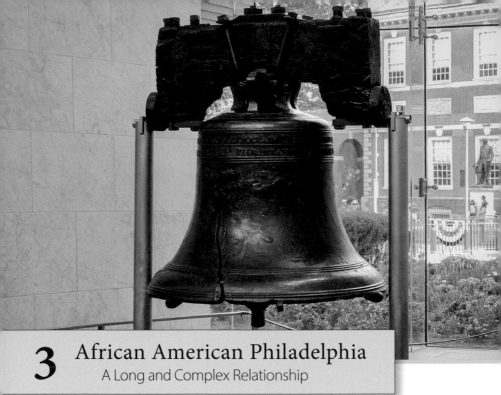

3 African American Philadelphia
A Long and Complex Relationship

Above: The Liberty Bell is an icon of independence and freedom, which is why abolitionists adopted it as a symbol.

BOUNDARIES: Arch St., South St., Front St., Seventh St.
DISTANCE: 2.4 miles
DIFFICULTY: Easy
PARKING: Metered parking is available along both South and Front Sts.
PUBLIC TRANSIT: SEPTA's 40 bus stops about three blocks away.

The first Africans in Philadelphia arrived in chains. Records show Dutch and Swedish settlers in the Delaware Valley imported enslaved Africans as early as 1639. The founder of the Commonwealth of Pennsylvania, William Penn, believed in equal rights for people of different religions, an anomaly for his time, but he also owned slaves.

But it was here in Philadelphia and in Pennsylvania that the earliest movements to break those chains began. The Germantown Quaker Petition Against Slavery, published in the city in

1688, was the colonies' first antislavery protest. Pennsylvania was the first state to pass a law ordering the emancipation of enslaved individuals within its borders.

This tour showcases people and places integral to African American history, beginning where Mason and Dixon began their land survey. It features sites where abolitionists worked, slaves took shelter, and freed African Americans made their marks.

Walk Description

Start at Front and South Streets, near I-95's overhead pedestrian crossing. Here, in 1763, Charles Mason and Jeremiah Dixon began surveying work to end a land dispute between William Penn and Baltimore's Calvert family. Mason and Dixon spent four years evaluating 244 miles of land, then created their "line." Less than a century later, this imaginary marker would divide free states from slave-holding states.

Turn left on Front Street. Walk four blocks north, paralleling the Delaware River. A sign marks where Thomas Paine founded the Society for the Relief of Free Negroes Unlawfully Held in Bondage in 1775. The organization became the Pennsylvania Abolition Society, and its president, Benjamin Franklin, petitioned the new US Congress to ban slavery. After the Civil War, the organization was a model for groups seeking equal opportunities for African Americans.

Cross Spruce Street. The ❶ **Philadelphia Korean War Memorial** at Penn's Landing contains details about the United States' role in the conflict between 1950 and 1953. In 1951, the all-Black 24th Infantry Regiment, which had served in the Spanish-American War and World Wars I and II, was disbanded, essentially ending segregation in the US Army. About 100,000 African American soldiers served in Korea at the start of the war—rising to more than 600,000 by the time it ended.

Continue north. At Walnut Street, look right toward the river where enslaved Jane Johnson and her two sons sought freedom in 1855. The three had been brought to Philadelphia from North Carolina by John Wheeler, who intended to take them overseas. Pennsylvania was a free state, and Johnson called for help, escaping with the help of two local abolitionists. One of the men was jailed, accused of kidnapping. Johnson, a fugitive who knew she could be arrested if she came back to Philadelphia, returned to refute that claim during the man's trial, testifying that she'd left willingly, adding "I would rather die than go back." The Johnsons settled in New England. One son served with the US Colored Troops during the Civil War.

Continue to Market Street. At right is a statue of Tamanend, chief of the native Lenni Lenape nation. His name is synonymous with affable, and settlers considered him their patron saint. Tamanend said the Lenni Lenape and the settlers would "live in peace as the waters run in the rivers and creeks and as long as the stars and moon endure."

The London Coffee House stood at the corner. Here, captured Africans were dragged from ships docked on the Delaware River and sold at auction. Census data from the 1760s shows one out of every six households had at least one slave. Thomas Paine wrote one of the first editorials condemning slavery while living in a nearby room.

Head west on Market Street. At ❷ **Franklin Fountain,** bow-tied staff serve homemade ice cream in a parlor with a 19th-century vibe. During a Black History Month celebration, a company blog post highlighted the role soda and ice-cream counters played in the Civil Rights movement. One of the country's first sit-ins was at Durham, North Carolina's Royal Ice Cream Parlor in 1957, when seven African Americans entered via the "Whites Only" entrance, sat in a booth, and ordered ice cream. Each was arrested and fined $10. They appealed, and theirs was the first court case challenging the legality of segregation.

Cross North Second Street and turn right. ❸ **Christ Church,** founded in 1695, hosted George Washington and other founders. It also has a role in early African American church history: Absalom Jones, the Episcopal Church's first African American priest, was ordained here. Jones also cofounded the Free African Society with Richard Allen and Cyrus Bustill.

Continue north. At Arch Street, turn left. ❹ **Cyrus Bustill's bakery** stood at 210 Arch Street. Born enslaved in 1732, Bustill was sold to a baker, who taught him his trade and then released him. Bustill baked bread for Washington's troops; he was one of 5,000 freed African Americans who aided the patriot cause. After the war, Bustill opened his bakery and was active in the Underground Railroad. Bustill's great, great-grandson was Civil Rights activist Paul Robeson.

Continue on Arch Street to the ❺ **Betsy Ross House,** where a reenactor plays Phillis, a freed African American who worked as a domestic in

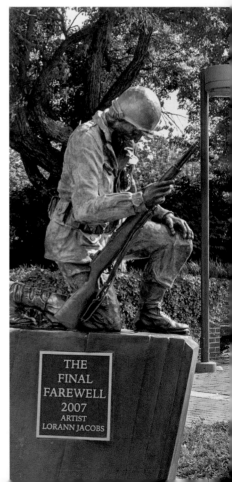

The Korean War memorial at Penn's Landing

THE
FINAL
FAREWELL
2007
ARTIST
LORANN JACOBS

Colonial Philadelphia. It's likely Ross hired someone like Phillis, as she was too busy running her upholstery shop to do housework.

Continue on Arch Street, crossing North Third Street. In 1775, Quaker leaders at the ❻ **Arch Street Meeting House** asked members to free their slaves. By 1778, most area Quakers had done so. The term *Quaker* was originally meant as an insult, referring to the way some members shook with emotion during services.

Continue to North Fifth and Arch Streets, passing Ben Franklin's grave. Cross Arch Street to the United States Mint, where the headquarters of the ❼ **Philadelphia Female Anti-Slavery Society** once stood. Founded in 1833 by Lucretia Mott and others, the society was interracial, enraging the pro-slavery crowd. Members sold baked goods, needlework, and pottery to raise money for causes, including the Underground Railroad. The society also ran a school for children of African descent and called for a boycott of products made with slave labor.

Continue on Arch Street, passing the Constitution Center and the Free Quaker Meeting House. Turn right on North Sixth Street. Public radio station WHYY's headquarters stands on the former site of ❽ **Pennsylvania Hall.** Financed by abolitionists seeking a safe meeting space, the hall formally opened on May 14, 1838. A letter from former president John Quincy Adams, read at the building's dedication, said, "I learnt with great satisfaction . . . that the Pennsylvania Hall Association have erected a large building in your city, wherein liberty and equality of civil rights can be freely discussed, and the evils of slavery fearlessly portrayed. . . . I rejoice that, in the city of Philadelphia, the friends of free discussion have erected a Hall for its unrestrained exercise." Four days after it opened, a mob burned the hall to the ground.

Return to Arch Street, continuing west. Across North Seventh Street is the ❾ **African American Museum,** founded in 1976. Its permanent collection includes more than 500,000 photos by Jack T. Franklin, who did work for *The Philadelphia Tribune,* the nation's oldest African American newspaper, and captured images during the 1963 March on Washington, the 1965 Selma to Montgomery March, and the first major Black Power rally in 1966. A sculpture outside honors Crispus Attucks, an escaped slave killed during 1770's Boston Massacre, the first casualty of the War for Independence.

Turn left on North Seventh Street, passing the Federal Detention Center (700 Arch St.). Museum officials initially opposed the building's construction, saying it would be a reminder of the African American community's disproportionate incarceration rates. Local businesses said the presence of prisoners would drive away customers. To appease critics, the facility, completed in 1997, is connected to the James A. Byrne US Courthouse via underground tunnel.

Continue south on North Seventh Street. The block-long Victorian structure before Market Street is actually 33 buildings, constructed between 1895 and 1907, with a common interior.

Now housing multiple businesses, this was the Lit Brothers Department Store, an affordable alternative to Wanamaker's. Its slogan: "A Great Store in a Great City." Lit's was known for its millinery department; the building's ghost signs still promise, "Hats Trimmed Free of Charge."

Cross Market Street. **⑩ Declaration House** is a reconstruction of the home where Thomas Jefferson rented a room while writing the Declaration of Independence. Jefferson's original draft contained a 168-word section condemning slavery as one of the evils of King George III who "waged cruel war against human nature itself, violating its most sacred rights of life & liberty in the persons of a distant people who never offended him, captivating & carrying them into slavery in another hemisphere," according to history.com. In Jefferson's autobiography, he blamed southern states for the removal of the passage but noted that northern states also had no wish to upset the status quo. Jefferson is thought to have enslaved more than 600 people during his lifetime, including the six children he fathered with Sally Hemings, a biracial woman born into slavery and believed to be the half-sister of Jefferson's wife, Martha.

Facing Declaration House, turn left, walking east. Stop at South Sixth Street. Across Market Street, on the south side of the Independence Visitor Center, is Alison Sky's *Indelible*. The work features sections from the Declaration of Independence, including the antislavery passage that was later removed. From certain angles, that passage is blurry, as if erased, forcing the viewer to move to see it clearly.

Cross South Sixth Street, renamed Avenue of Freedom in 2019 to mark key events in African American history. (Intersecting Market Street was rechristened "Avenue of Our Founders" at the same time.)

The first White House features an exhibit remembering enslaved people who worked there.

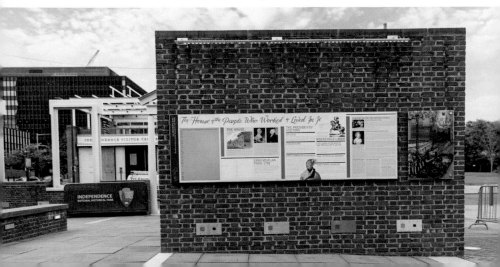

⓫ **The President's House** was the nation's first executive mansion, home to Presidents George Washington and John Quincy Adams. The exhibit remembers the nine slaves Washington kept here. (His letters show he went to great lengths to subvert a Pennsylvania law that freed slaves who lived in the city for an unbroken six-month stretch by sending them on day trips to New Jersey.) Among the enslaved was Oney Judge, a gifted seamstress who was Martha Washington's personal maid. Judge escaped. Washington twice sent mercenaries to recapture her. Twice they failed. She was still considered a fugitive when she died more than 50 years later.

Turn right, heading south on South Sixth Street, passing the ⓬ **Liberty Bell Pavilion.** The bell, commissioned in 1751, is inscribed with the Biblical quote, "Proclaim Liberty throughout all the land unto all the inhabitants thereof." Before the 1830s, Philadelphians called it the old bell. Then abolitionists adopted it as a symbol of their movement, and New York Anti-Slavery Society dubbed it the Liberty Bell, telling their Philadelphia counterparts, "the bell has not obeyed the inscription and its peals have been a mockery, when one sixth of 'all inhabitants' are in abject slavery."

Continue south, crossing Chestnut Street, to Independence Hall. In the 1800s, recaptured slaves went on trial here. An 1851 newspaper article details the case of "two alleged fugitives, Helen and Dick." One man testified that, "Helen had been his slave; his father had owned her mother Charity, whose mother he had bought they were made a present about six months after the marriage."

Across South Sixth Street is the Public Ledger Building, the former headquarters of the city's first "penny paper," which began publishing in 1836. (Most newspapers cost a nickel at the time.) The paper's motto was "Virtue Liberty and Independence." The editorial staff favored abolition.

Continue south, crossing Walnut Street, here called World Heritage Way. The Penn Mutual Tower (510 Walnut St.) rises where the Walnut Street Prison stood from 1775 to 1835. Before that, Reverend Richard Allen, a former slave turned minister, had a blacksmith shop here. Allen moved the shop to land he owned at South Sixth and Lombard Streets, where he founded the country's first African Methodist Episcopal Church.

Across South Sixth Street is ⓭ **Washington Square,** one of the city's five original green spaces. In early days, this was a graveyard for slaves and the very poor and a popular gathering place for enslaved Africans, earning it the name Congo Square. During the Revolutionary War, soldiers from both sides were interred here, prompting John Adams in 1777 to say the graves "are enough to make the heart of stone melt away." The square also holds victims of disease outbreaks, including the 1793 yellow fever epidemic. The Tomb of the Unknown Revolutionary War soldier is marked by a statue of George Washington and an eternal flame.

Continue south on South Sixth Street. **⑭ Athenaeum of Philadelphia,** a member-supported museum and library, is the go-to resource for information about architecture and interior design from 1800 to 1945.

Continue to Spruce Street. Holy Trinity Church was built in 1789 by the city's German Catholic community. In 1797, the church opened the country's first Catholic orphanage for children whose parents died from yellow fever.

Cross Spruce Street. The building on the right was the home of actor Joseph Jefferson (1829–1905), one of the most famous comedians of his time. He was four when he went on stage for the first time, in black face, with an adult actor playing a character called "Jim Crow."

The historically designated home at 538–540 Spruce Street was for sale in 2021 for $1.95 million. This neighborhood has one of the country's largest concentrations of original 18th- and 19th-century buildings.

Continue south. **⑮ Mother Bethel African Methodist Episcopal Church** was founded in 1794 by Richard Allen, mentioned earlier. This is the world's first A.M.E. church, sitting on the oldest parcel of land in the United States continuously owned by African Americans. Original congregants came here because of forced segregation at other churches. A devoted abolitionist, Allen began helping newly freed slaves arriving in the city in the 1790s. The church became part of the Underground Railroad.

The current church, built in the late 1800s, includes a museum with items belonging to the 2,500 black soldiers Allen rallied to fight in the War of 1812. Allen, who died in 1831, is entombed here. One admirer called him "one of the greatest divines who has lived since the apostolic age."

At South Sixth and Lombard Streets, a marker refers to the 1842 Lombard Street riot. On August 1, about 1,000 members of an all-Black abolitionist group paraded to commemorate the anniversary of slavery's end in the West Indies, carrying a banner reading "How grand in age, how fair in truth, are holy Friendship, Love and Truth." There'd been low-simmering tension between Irish Catholic immigrants and the freed African Americans as they competed for jobs and housing. During three days of conflict, one church was burned down and several homes were looted.

Continue to South Street. Turn right to see *Mapping Courage: Honoring W. E. B. Du Bois and Engine #11.* Du Bois, a Harvard University PhD, conducted a door-to-door survey of African Americans. His research resulted in *The Philadelphia Negro.* Du Bois famously asked, "Would America have been America without her Negro people?"

Engine #11 was the city's first and only fire company composed of African American firefighters, who were known as "leather lungs" because they took on the most dangerous blazes. The Philadelphia Fire Department was desegregated in 1952.

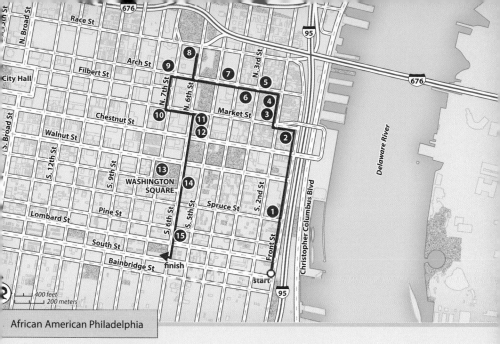

Points of Interest

① **Philadelphia Korean War Memorial** Penn's Landing, between Dock and Spruce Sts.

② **Franklin Fountain** 116 Market St., 215-627-1899, franklinfountain.com

③ **Christ Church** 20 N. American St., 215-922-1695, christchurchphila.org

④ **Cyrus Bustill's bakery** 210 Arch St. (not open to the public)

⑤ **Betsy Ross House** 239 Arch St., 215-629-4026, historicphiladelphia.org/what-to-see

⑥ **Arch Street Meeting House** 320 Arch St., 215-413-1804, historicasmh.org

⑦ **Philadelphia Female Anti-Slavery Society (now the United States Mint)** 151 N. Independence Mall E., 215-408-0112, usmint.com

⑧ **Former site of Pennsylvania Hall (now WHYY headquarters)** 150 N. Sixth St., 215-351-1200, whyy.org

⑨ **African American Museum** 701 Arch St., 215-574-0380, aampmuseum.org

⑩ **Declaration House** 599 S. Seventh St., 215-965-2305, nps.gov/inde

⑪ **The President's House** 524–30 Market St., 800-537-7676, phlvisitorcenter.com

⑫ **Liberty Bell Pavilion** S. Sixth and Market Sts., 215-965-2305, nps.gov/inde

⑬ **Washington Square** Walnut St. between Sixth and Seventh Sts., 215-965-2305, nps.gov/inde

⑭ **Athenaeum of Philadelphia** 219 S. Sixth St., 215-925-2688, philaathenaeum.org

⑮ **Mother Bethel African Methodist Episcopal Church** 419 S. Sixth St., 215-925-0616, motherbethel.org

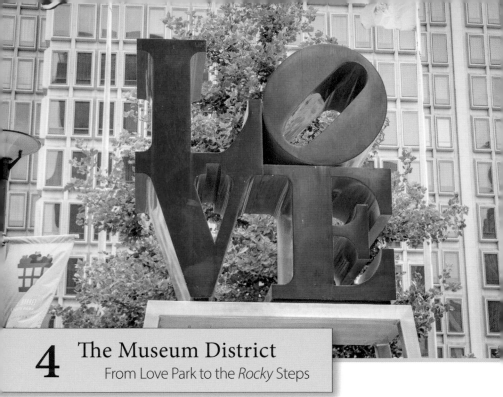

4 The Museum District
From Love Park to the *Rocky* Steps

Above: One of pop artist Robert Indiana's Love statues, located in a park by City Hall, is perfect for The City of Brotherly Love.

BOUNDARIES: N. 15th St., N. 24th St., Arch St., Kelly Dr.
DISTANCE: A direct walk from Love Park to The Philadelphia Museum of Art is 1 mile. Figure another 0.5 mile for your detours.
DIFFICULTY: Easy
PARKING: Street parking is very limited in this neighborhood, as are public parking lots. Public transportation is the best way to get here.
PUBLIC TRANSIT: Options include taking the SEPTA Market–Frankford or Broad Street Line; any regional rail line; or bus routes including 2, 17, 27, 31, 32, 33, 44, 124, and 125.

Benjamin Franklin Parkway is one of the country's earliest examples of urban renewal, a marked departure from William Penn's grid. This 1-mile stretch has been called Philadelphia's Champs-Élysées, running through its cultural heart. In a downtown of narrow streets and alleys, some impassable by cars, the parkway stands out.

Walk Description

Start at John F. Kennedy Plaza, at 15th Street and John F. Kennedy Boulevard, better known as ❶ **Love Park** because of pop artist Robert Indiana's iconic red sculpture. Versions of this 1950s work are in cities worldwide, including New York, Indianapolis, and Tokyo.

The fountain honors local philanthropist Ellen Phillips Samuel. City leaders dye the fountain's water to mark specific events, such as pink for Breast Cancer Awareness Month. A less popular case: the water flowed blood red in 2007 to promote Showtime's *Dexter,* about a serial killer who kills serial killers.

Love Park, opened in 1965, was the brainchild of city planner Edmund Bacon, whose influence is seen throughout Philadelphia. In 2002, when officials talked of banning skateboards in the park, the 92-year-old Bacon strapped on a helmet and, with the help of aides, rolled through. He later said, "My whole damn life has been worth it, just for this."

Walk west on John F. Kennedy Boulevard toward the glass building that looks like a flying saucer. The ❷ **Love Park Welcome Center** is one of Center City's best examples of mid-century modern architecture. It opened in 1960 as the Philadelphia Hospitality Center. A multimillion-dollar renovation, expected to be completed by late 2022, will add a restaurant and outdoor seating.

Across from the saucer stands Suburban Station (16th St. and JFK Blvd.). When the Art Deco building opened in 1930 for "electrified train operation," about 56,000 people used the trains for daily commutes.

Cross 16th Street and turn right. Cross Arch Street. *Monument to Six Million Jewish Martyrs,* placed in 1964, was a gift from a group whose families fled Europe during World War II. It was the country's first public monument to Holocaust victims. Polish-born sculptor Nathan Rapoport created about a dozen other Holocaust memorials, the most famous being *Memorial to the Warsaw Ghetto Uprising.*

Walk northwest along Benjamin Franklin Parkway. Flags representing 90 nations, installed in 1976, celebrate the city's diversity. In 2022, after

Academy of Natural Sciences scientist Ted Daeschler co-discovered Tiktaalik roseae, the fossil believed to show the link between fish and land animals.

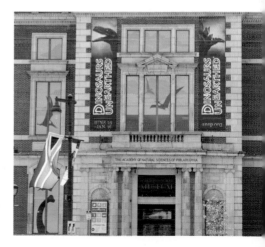

Russia invaded Ukraine, city officials reported multiple thefts of the Russian flag. In summer 2022, a petition permanently removing the Russian flag was in circulation.

Tuscan Girl (1776 Ben Franklin Pkwy.) is a nonworking fountain, installed in 1965 as part of a program requiring developers to spend 1% of their construction budget on public art. It's unclear which figure is the Tuscan girl.

Cross 18th Street. The statue of General Thaddeus Kosciuszko honors the Polish-born engineer who showed revolutionaries how to strengthen their waterfront positions. He also helped build West Point, New York's fortification, later called the American Gibraltar.

Because of the parkway's width, crossing as a pedestrian can be a challenge. To reach ❸ **Sister Cities Park,** walk to the Swedish flag, use the crosswalk to reach the median, then cross again to reach the far side of the parkway.

Dedicated in 1976, Sister Cities was neglected for decades before a 2012 renovation added climbing rocks, a cafe, and a boat pond. The 1.75-acre park's centerpiece is a fountain with Philadelphia at the center, surrounded by spouts representing its 10 sister cities. Robert Indiana's 6-foot-tall *AMOR*, which means "love" in Spanish and Latin, was acquired for Pope Francis's 2015 visit.

Logan Square, a popular gathering place, features the Swann Fountain.

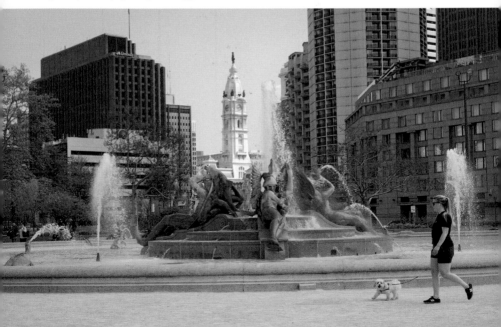

Two statues here honor European-born men who were essential to the patriots' cause: Irish immigrant Thomas Fitzsimons funded Washington's army and later served three Congressional terms. Don Diego de Gardoqui, the first US ambassador to Spain, secured funds from Spanish banks.

Follow the diagonal path northwest to the corner of Vine Street and the parkway. Turn left. Take the crosswalk under the Botswana flag to the median, then follow the next crosswalk to ❹ **Logan Square,** one of the city's five original green spaces. The square hosted public executions in the 1700s and public gatherings in the 1800s, including 1864's Great Sanitary Fair, which raised funds for bandages and other medical items for Union soldiers. The Swann Memorial Fountain, installed in 1924, was designed by Alexander Stirling Calder, whose father's statue of William Penn tops City Hall and whose son crafted another nearby work. The three bronze Native Americans represent the city's three main waterways: The Delaware and Schuylkill Rivers and Wissahickon Creek. The water-spouting swans are a pun on the fountain's name, which honors Wilson Cary Swann, the first president of the Philadelphia Fountain Society, which installed public water fountains for humans and animals.

Walk three-quarters of the way around the fountain, then cross the parkway to the ❺ **Academy of Natural Sciences of Drexel University.** Founded in 1812 by some of the country's leading naturalists, this is the oldest natural-sciences institution in the Western Hemisphere, housed here since 1876.

The statue closest to the door shows two small, meat-eating dinosaurs reminiscent of *Jurassic Park*'s velociraptors. These are *Deinonychus,* which means "terrible claw." The other statue is Joseph Leidy, the father of American vertebrate paleontology. He holds the jawbone of the Ice Age lion he identified.

Turn right onto Race Street. ❻ **Moore College of Art & Design** is the county's first and only all-female college of art and design. Its gallery is public.

Continue to 20th Street and turn right. ❼ **Aviator Park** features Paul Manship's *Aero Memorial*, a monument to World War I pilots. The celestial sphere shows the constellations and the signs of the zodiac. The artist included a carving of himself with a star on his forehead near the Pisces sign.

Turn left and walk around the low wall. *All Wars Memorial to Colored Soldiers and Sailors* depicts real fighters who posed for the artist. Completed in 1934, when the US military was still segregated, the monument was initially placed in an obscure corner of Fairmount Park. It moved here in 1994, almost 50 years after President Harry S. Truman's executive order integrated the military.

At the corner of 20th and Winter Streets, turn left, crossing 20th Street. Founded in 1824 and named for Ben Franklin, ❽ **The Franklin Institute** is one of the nation's premier museums, as well as a center for science education and research. The institute accepted its first female scientist for membership in 1833; the first member of African descent was welcomed in 1870. Among the museum's permanent exhibitions are the *Giant Heart* and *Your Brain*. The national monument to Franklin, in the museum's rotunda, features a 20-foot-tall, 30-ton sculpture of the Founding Father.

The institute's scientists are highly respected, so citizens panicked in March 1940 when a local radio station reported the world would end the next day, April 1, as "confirmed by astronomers of The Franklin Institute, Philadelphia." The station had learned of Earth's imminent doom from an institute press release, which specifically noted this was *not* an April Fool's Day joke. It was.

Continue on Winter Street. At 21st Street, turn right. Follow the Vine Street Expressway crosswalk to return to the parkway.

Turn left, crossing 22nd Street, and continue toward 24th Street. The green space below you on the left is Paine's Skateboard Park (Martin Luther King Jr. and Benjamin Franklin Pkwys.), which opened in 2013 as an outlet for skateboard enthusiasts.

At 24th Street, cross to the right median, then cross again to reach the square opposite the art museum.

❾ Eakins Oval, the "Park on the Parkway," is 8 acres of public space named for painter Thomas Eakins. It has been center stage for numerous events, including Masses led by Pope John Paul II in 1979 and Pope Francis in 2015, 2005's Live 8 Concert, and the city's annual Fourth of July concerts. The largest fountain features George Washington astride a horse. The artist modeled the face on a mask made during Washington's lifetime.

Leave the oval via the walkway nearest the corner of Kelly Drive and the parkway. Cross the street at the crosswalk.

Walk left to the steps of the **❿ Philadelphia Museum of Art.** Built in 1928, the museum is not only one of the largest in the country—with works by Henri Matisse, Marcel Duchamp, Paul Cézanne, and John Singer Sargent—but also a well-known movie location. Many visitors charge the steps, as seen in three of the *Rocky* films. In 2011, screenjunkies.com said the steps were the world's second-most-famous movie location. (Grand Central Terminal was first.) To the right of the steps is a statue of fictional boxer Rocky Balboa, originally a movie prop.

Pass Rocky to reach *Charioteer of Delphi,* a bronze cast of an original 5th-century BC work, a gift from the Greek government in 1976. The final stop, *Young Meher,* is a memorial to the thousands of Armenians killed by the Ottoman Empire in 1915, gifted to the city by the local Armenian community. Meher, an Armenian folk hero from the Middle Ages, looks skyward, holding a cross aloft as he prepares for battle.

The second parkway tour (page 28) returns to Love Park.

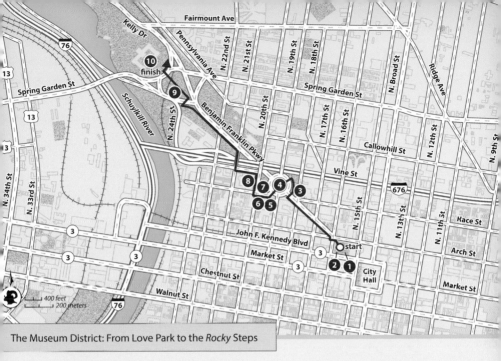

The Museum District: From Love Park to the *Rocky* Steps

Points of Interest

① **Love Park** 15th St. and John F. Kennedy Blvd.

② **Love Park Welcome Center** 1599 John F. Kennedy Blvd., 215-344 8544,
phlvisitorcenter.com/lovepark

③ **Sister Cities Park** 218 N. 18th St., 215-440-5500, centercityphila.org/parks/sister-cities-park

④ **Logan Square** Vine Street Expressway and Benjamin Franklin Parkway,
tinyurl.com/logansquarephilly

⑤ **Academy of Natural Sciences of Drexel University** 1900 Benjamin Franklin Parkway,
215-299-1000, ansp.org

⑥ **Moore College of Art & Design** 1916 Race St., 215-965-4000, moore.edu

⑦ **Aviator Park** Race and N. 20th Sts.

⑧ **The Franklin Institute** 222 N. 20th St., 215-448-1200, fi.edu

⑨ **Eakins Oval** 2451 Benjamin Franklin Parkway, 215-607-3477, theovalphl.org

⑩ **Philadelphia Museum of Art** 2600 Benjamin Franklin Parkway, 215-763-8100, philamuseum.org

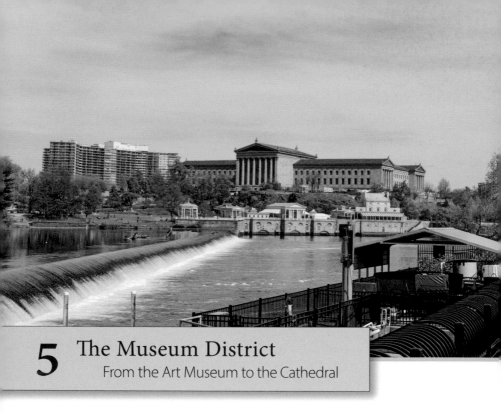

5 The Museum District
From the Art Museum to the Cathedral

BOUNDARIES: Fairmount Ave., Ben Franklin Pkwy., Pennsylvania Ave., N. 16th St.
DISTANCE: About 2 miles, depending on how many detours you take
DIFFICULTY: Easy. It's a flat walk.
PARKING: There is a parking garage behind the building that you can reach via Art Museum Drive or Waterworks Drive.
PUBLIC TRANSIT: SEPTA bus routes 2, 7, 32, 33, and 48, or take the PHLASH to Stop 13.

This walk covers the north side of Benjamin Franklin Parkway and includes some of the city's most popular museums and some of the amazing statuary that makes Philadelphia an outdoor art gallery. It ends at Love Park.

Walk Description

Begin at the art museum's ❶ **Ruth and Raymond G. Perelman Building,** at Fairmount and Pennsylvania Avenues. This Art Deco structure, built in 1926, was the headquarters for Fidelity Mutual Life Insurance Company. Look for Egyptian-style sculptures of animals representing the attributes of insurance: the opossum of protection, the owl of wisdom, the dog of fidelity, the pelican of charity, and the squirrel of frugality.

The words above the Pennsylvania Avenue entrance read: "In the honor and perpetuity of the family is founded the state. In the nobler life of the household is the nobler life of mankind."

Begin walking southeast on Pennsylvania Avenue. At 25th Street, turn right. The golden *Joan of Arc* statue (Kelly Dr. and 25th St.) shows the medieval French heroine astride a horse and ready to fight the English during the Hundred Years' War. Two other casts of Emmanuel Frémiet's original 1874 statue are displayed in Portland, Oregon, and New Orleans. Some locals call this "Joanie on a pony."

Follow Kelly Drive to *Symbiosis* (24th St. and Kelly Dr.), a 34-foot-tall shimmering silver sculpture installed in 2014. Artist Roxy Paine hand-soldered thousands of pieces of stainless steel pipes, plates, and rods to create what could be a tree or a part of the vascular system. Nearby is *Iroquois* (Benjamin Franklin Pkwy. at Eakins Oval and Spring Garden St.), a 40-foot-tall red steel sculpture installed in 2007. Abstract impressionist sculptor Mark di Suvero describes his works, made of steel I beams, as "paintings in three dimensions with the crane as my paintbrush."

Continue east, passing Von Colln Memorial Park, named for Philadelphia Police Department Sergeant Frank Von Colln, killed on duty in August 1970.

Some visitors are confused to see a copy of Auguste Rodin's *The Thinker* here, but Philadelphia has the largest collection of Rodin's works outside of Paris. The ❷ **Rodin Museum's** collection was a gift from movie theater magnate Jules Mastbaum. He died before it opened in 1929.

The museum honors the artist's French roots with a formal French garden on-site. The building is a scaled-down version of a grand Beaux Arts structure. As noted in the first parkway tour (page 22), the parkway's original architects envisioned it as a grand boulevard, like Paris's Champs-Élysées.

Next is the ❸ **Barnes Foundation,** which houses the extensive art collection of self-made millionaire Dr. Albert Barnes. In 1922, Barnes opened his museum in the suburb of Lower Merion, personally placing each work of art—including pieces by Renoir, Matisse, Picasso, Cézanne, and Seurat—in exhibition rooms that highlighted the relationship between the objects.

Barnes died in 1951, and his will decreed the museum remain in the suburbs. The controversial move to downtown Philadelphia was completed in 2012. Supporters note more than 1 million people visited the Philadelphia location in one year, almost three times the number of visitors who went to the suburban location in five years.

The museum is a low-key, two-storied limestone structure some have called sophisticated, simple, and soulful. Inside, the art is displayed in rooms that are almost exact replicas of the ones Barnes himself decorated.

Continue toward 20th Street. Keep straight, ignoring the parkway's bend. The road becomes Vine Street. The ❹ **Free Library of Philadelphia**, the cornerstone of the city's public library system, opened in 1927.

Ben Franklin created the country's first library system when he and 50 friends combined funds to buy books for the new Library Company. Years later, Franklin noted that foreign visitors were impressed by Philadelphians' sophistication, which they credited to the locals' love of reading.

The neighboring building at 1801 Vine Street, a New Deal public works project built in 1938, once housed the municipal court system's juvenile and domestic branches. Its exterior reveals

The Cathedral Basilica of Saints Peter & Paul is the principal church of the Archdiocese of Philadelphia. Pope Francis performed Mass here in 2015.

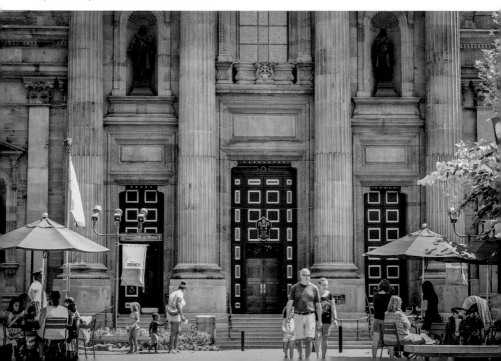

its original intentions. Note the two triangular pediments on the upper front corners. At left is *Juvenile Protection,* which includes a seated woman with an olive branch sitting near the scales of justice. At right is *Family Unity,* which shows a reclining woman holding a baby and a reclining man holding a dog.

Continue on Vine Street. Completed in 2016, ❺ **The Church of Jesus Christ of Latter-day Saints** is the local home for 41,000 Mormon faithful. The 197-foot-tall white structure is topped with a gold-leafed Angel Moroni, who led founder Joseph Smith to the golden plates from which *The Book of Mormon* was derived. The temple, open only to Mormons, is used for special ceremonies. The building across the street is for regular worship.

Circle the building to fully appreciate its size, then return to 18th Street and cross the road. ❻ **Cathedral Basilica of Saints Peter & Paul** (18th and Race Sts.) is the principal church of the Catholic Archdiocese of Philadelphia. Completed in 1864, it's modeled after Rome's Church of Saint Charles. It originally had no street-level windows for fear of vandalism after the anti-Catholic riots in the 1840s. To determine window placement, the architect tossed rocks at the building, then placed the windows above the highest rock strike. Lower windows were added during a 1950s renovation.

To the right is *Jesus Breaking Bread,* depicting a young Christ holding a broken half of pita bread in each hand. This sculpture caused a stir in 1976, with critics claiming artist Walter Erlebacher's depiction of Christ was inaccurate. (The artist's response: How do you know? Do you have photos?) Supporters said the statue seems to be calling people to church.

Continue to the corner of Benjamin Franklin Parkway and turn left. *Three Disks, One Lacking* is by Alexander Calder of the great Calder family of artists. His grandfather is perhaps best known for the William Penn statue atop City Hall, while his father designed Logan Square's Swann Memorial Fountain; both are visible from here. Look through the sculpture's cutout section. The William Penn statue atop City Hall is perfectly framed within the loop.

Continue to Henry Moore's *Three Way Piece Number One: Points* between 16th and 17th Streets. Installed in 1990, this bronze statue on a black-granite base changes as viewers circle it. The artist said "sculpture should always at first sight have some obscurities and further meanings." Some people see a three-legged animal; others, a giant tooth.

Continue to 16th Street. Jacob Lipkin's *The Prophet* is at the corner. Ahead is Love Park. Consider a stop at ❼ **Capriccio at Café Cret,** a small coffee bar named after French-born architect Paul Philippe Cret, one of the parkway's principal planners.

This tour ends here. Continue to City Hall to pick up another tour (Walk 8, page 46).

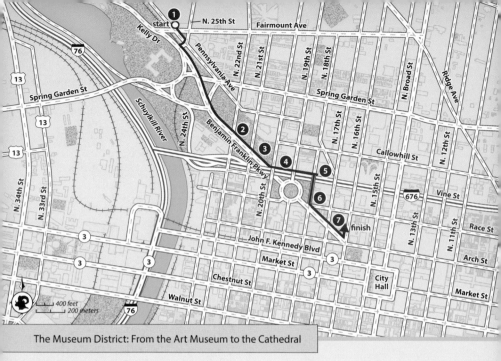

The Museum District: From the Art Museum to the Cathedral

Points of Interest

1 **Ruth and Raymond G. Perelman Building** Fairmount and Pennsylvania Aves., 215-763-8100, philamuseum.org

2 **Rodin Museum** 2151 Benjamin Franklin Parkway, 215-763-8100, rodinmuseum.org

3 **Barnes Foundation** 2025 Benjamin Franklin Parkway, 215-278-7000, barnesfoundation.org

4 **Free Library of Philadelphia** 1901 Vine St., 833-TALK-FLP (825-5357), freelibrary.org

5 **The Church of Jesus Christ of Latter-day Saints** 1739 Vine St., 215-398-3040, lds.org/church/temples

6 **Cathedral Basilica of Saints Peter & Paul** 1723 Race St., 215-561-1313, cathedralphila.org

7 **Capriccio at Café Cret** N. 16th St. and Benjamin Franklin Parkway 215-735-9797, capricciocafe.com

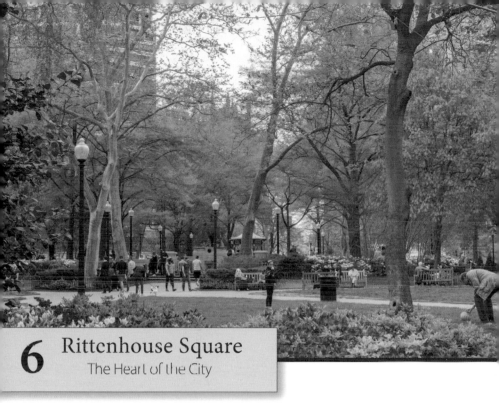

6 Rittenhouse Square
The Heart of the City

Above: Rittenhouse Square is the city's busiest downtown park.

BOUNDARIES: S. 17th St., S. 20th St., Delancey Pl., Walnut St.
DISTANCE: 1.1 miles
DIFFICULTY: Easy
PARKING: Street parking is a challenge near Rittenhouse, and the few paid lots are overpriced. Public transportation may be the best option.
PUBLIC TRANSIT: SEPTA buses 9, 12, 21, and 42 stopping on Walnut St. The SEPTA subway stop is at 19th and Market Sts., two blocks north of the square.

Rittenhouse Square is one of the city's five original squares, part of William Penn's plan for a "greene country town." The park was once lined with single-family mansions designed by the city's most illustrious architects. In 1953's *Gentlemen Prefer Blondes,* Marilyn Monroe sang, "A house on Rittenhouse Square wouldn't be so hard to take."

Today, only four of these mansions remain, most replaced by high-end, high-rise residences and hotels. A popular meeting place for locals, the square is constantly bustling and offers great people-watching. It hosts an annual art fair, weekly farmers markets, and occasional concerts. In 2010, the American Planning Association included Rittenhouse on its list of the country's top 10 Great Public Spaces. That's ironic, as in the 1700s the square was a pasture for livestock and for dumping "night soils." It was cleaned and renamed for astronomer David Rittenhouse in 1825.

Walk Description

Begin at South 18th and Manning Streets. The nonprofit Philadelphia Art Alliance (251 S. 18th St.) was founded in 1915 to present a variety of art forms in one venue. It features up to 12 exhibitions a year. It is housed in the former Wetherill mansion, one of only four residential properties still standing.

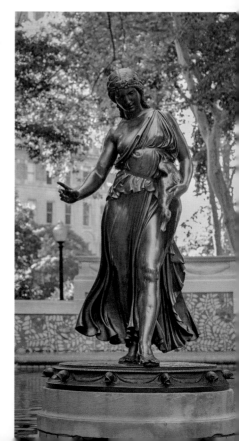

Walk north on South 18th Street. Cross Stowkowski Place, named for conductor Leopold Stowkowski, who proposed *Fantasia* to Walt Disney and then led the Philadelphia Orchestra through seven of the film's eight musical segments.

At left is ❶ **Rittenhouse Square**. At right, the former Barclay Hotel (237 S. 18th St.) was the finest hotel in the city when it opened in 1929. It became condominiums in 2005. Unit 6B—a 4,000-square-foot space with 3 bedrooms and 4 baths—was for sale in 2022 for $2.9 million. The monthly $3,000 dues include access to a chauffeur-driven 2019 Mercedes S-450.

Continue to the ❷ **Curtis Institute of Music,** which boasts that 30% of its graduates play with one of the country's "big five" orchestras. Notable alums include Leonard Bernstein and Samuel Barber. Curtis provides full-tuition, merit-based scholarships to all students. Its building was the

Paul Manship's Duck Girl *in Rittenhouse Square*

home of George Drexel, whose grandfather founded Drexel University. Drexel was the owner and editor of the *Philadelphia Public Ledger,* which high society considered "the only newspaper any lady or gentleman should read."

Turn right on Locust Street to appreciate the Curtis's architecture. A marker remembers Philadelphia-born Vincent Persichetti, a 1939 Curtis graduate who wrote nine symphonies.

Cross tiny Mozart Place, looking right to see Schubert Lane, then continuing on Locust. The commercial building at 1704 Locust Street is the headquarters of the Vidocq Society, a members-only organization that helps US law enforcement agencies investigate cold case homicides.

At South 17th Street, turn left. Pass the 20-story Warwick Hotel (1701 Locust St.), which was built in 1925 and has hosted four NFL drafts. Continue to Walnut Street. Before turning left, look at the architecture of 1701 Walnut Street, built in 1910 for the Estey Piano & Organ Company.

Continue west on Walnut Street. Two other buildings worth a second look are 1707 and 1709, originally private residences.

At South 18th Street, cross the road and enter Rittenhouse Square. Straight ahead is the Evelyn Taylor Price Memorial Sundial, installed in 1947, honoring a past president of the park-improvement association. One art historian called the statue—which features two children holding a sunflower—a "poetical reminder of the fleeting joys of sunshine."

Take the right path, passing *Giant Frog,* which is . . . a giant frog. Continue to the guardhouse, then turn right to the cluster of greenery holding a statue of a lion crushing a serpent. This is . . . *Lion Crushing Serpent,* a bronze cast of the original displayed in the Louvre. It's an allegory for the French Revolution, the lion symbolizing good and the serpent representing evil.

Turn around, passing the guardhouse, to reach Rittenhouse Fountain, designed by Benjamin Franklin Parkway architect Paul Phillipe Cret. Emerging from the water is Paul Manship's *Duck Girl,* a local favorite.

Continue straight. Descend four stairs and then turn right, following the curving, bench-lined walkway to *Billy,* another local landmark. The goat's horns have been rubbed to a shine because doing so is said to bring good luck. It's unclear why the tail has the same luster.

Follow Billy's right horn to exit onto Rittenhouse Square West. Turn left. Stop at the corner entrance, where *Rittenhouse Square Dogs* once stood (only one dog remains). The art was donated in 1988 by friends of late art collector Henry McIlhenny, whom Andy Warhol once called "the only person in Philadelphia with glamour."

Look right at 1914–16 Rittenhouse Square West. McIlhenny purchased six lots in 1950 and combined them to create the existing 8,600-square-foot structure. McIlhenny, a Philadelphia

Museum of Art curator and one-time chairman of its board, bequeathed his art collection—which included works by Degas, Toulouse-Lautrec, and Renoir—to the museum.

Ahead is the Philadelphia Ethical Society, 1906 Rittenhouse Square. The Ethical Culture movement is a non-theist alternative to traditional religion, established here in 1885.

Turn left on Rittenhouse Square South, then turn right on South 19th Street. Pass ❸ **Metropolitan Bakery,** a local favorite. At Spruce Street, turn left.

At the corner of South 18th Street sits the Gothic Revival ❹ **Temple Beth Zion–Beth Israel Synagogue**, built for a Methodist congregation but repurposed in 1954. Renovations included installing stained glass windows depicting important scenes from Jewish history and worship.

Cross South 18th Street. Most of the mansions on this block have been converted to condominiums or rental units. Continue to 1710 Spruce Street, the former home of the eccentric Harry K. Thaw, an heir to a Pittsburgh mine and railroad fortune who lit cigars with $5 bills. In 1906, Thaw shot and killed architect Stanford White in New York. Thaw's wife, actress Evelyn Nesbit, had previously dated White, which Thaw believed tainted her. His murder trial was the original trial of the century. Thaw was found not guilty by reason of insanity. E. L. Doctorow included the case in *Ragtime*.

At South 17th Street, turn right. At Delancey Place (also called Delancey Street), turn right again. ❺ **Plays and Players** is one of the oldest professional theater companies in the country. Actor Kevin Bacon appeared onstage here as a child in 1974.

At S. 18th Street, turn left. The single-family home at 1801 Delancey Street was built in 1857 for Mary Morris Husband, a Civil War nurse and granddaughter of Robert Morris, financier of the American Revolution. Her two sons were Union soldiers.

The home's current owners have kept a gladiator statue in their ground floor bay window since 2012. "Mr. 1801" changes clothes as appropriate, such as a cap and gown in May. A November 2020 post on Mr. 1801's 800-fan-strong Facebook page shows him draped in an American flag with a card that says, "Thank you, Philadelphia. Democracy won!"

Continue on Delancey Street. The homes at 1804 and 1806 have firemarks with a tree image. Homeowners with fire insurance displayed these medallions on their property's exterior to tell firefighters which insurance company would pay them. These tree marks were issued by Mutual Assurance of Philadelphia, aka The Green Tree Company, in the 1820s. Its symbol acknowledged that the company insured properties near trees, which others did not.

Continue west, passing 1813 Delancey, a 5,000-square-foot home with a roof deck, a gym, and garage parking that sold for $2.8 million in 2015. The private residence at 1827 Delancey Place, with a curved brick facade and an iron balcony, was built in 1861, but it has some distinctly modern touches, including an elevator and a working waterfall. In 2021, its estimated value was $3.4 million.

Continue west. General George Gordon Meade, who led Union forces to victory during 1863's Battle of Gettysburg, lived at 1836 Delancey Place and died here in 1872. This home was his reward, and his name remains engraved above the door.

Cross South 19th Street. The ❻ **Horace Jayne House** was designed by Frank Furness, who one critic noted "pushed ugliness to the point where it almost turned to beauty." The National Register of Historic Places says the design anticipates the work of Frank Lloyd Wright while recalling Thomas Jefferson's Monticello.

At South 19th Street, turn right. At Spruce Street, turn left. The ❼ **Rafsnyder-Welsh House** is a visual delight—or nightmare, depending on taste. Built in 1855 as a flat-roofed, redbrick home like neighboring structures, an 1890 renovation added red sandstone and terra-cotta trim. Note the different window shapes and the off-center entrance. The redesign inspired other homeowners to remodel similarly.

Continue on Spruce Street. At South 20th Street, turn left, then make a right on Delancey. These Civil War–era mansions remain largely unchanged. The block, one of the city's most picturesque residential stretches, is also its most filmed, featured in at least five movies or TV shows. In 1983's *Trading Places*, Dan Aykroyd's character lived at 2014 Delancey Place. In a scene from 1999's *The Sixth Sense*, Bruce Willis's character stands outside "his" house at 2006 Delancey Place.

The ❽ **Rosenbach Museum and Library** showcases the collections of Phillip and A. S. W. Rosenbach, dealers of rare books and manuscripts, in their former home. It includes letters written by Presidents George Washington and Abraham Lincoln, the only known surviving edition of Ben Franklin's original *Poor Richard's Almanack*, and Lewis Carroll's own copy of *Alice*

The Rafsnyder-Welsh House is a visual delight— or nightmare.

in Wonderland. The museum has James Joyce's handwritten *Ulysses* manuscript and celebrates the masterpiece annually on Bloomsday, June 16.

At South 21st Street, turn right. The property at 1752 has a firemark showing four hands holding the others' wrists in a box shape, meaning it was insured by Benjamin Franklin's The Philadelphia Contributionship, the country's oldest property insurance company, established in 1752.

Continue north. At Locust Street, turn right. Some mansions here have been converted into condominiums and apartments.

Cross South 20th Street. At Rittenhouse Square West, turn left. **9 The Rittenhouse** is a luxury hotel-residence featuring La Croix restaurant, which hosts a weekly $75-per-person Sunday brunch buffet called "the granddaddy of all Philly brunch spots" by *Philadelphia.* Dinner options include caviar tasting menus starting at $85.

The **10 Church of the Holy Trinity** dates to 1857 and has Tiffany stained glass windows. The bell tower rings hourly. In the 1860s, the church's rector wrote "O Little Town of Bethlehem."

At Walnut Street, turn right. Near the block's end, look left at 1811 Walnut Street, built for the Rittenhouse Club, an exclusive men's organization founded in 1874. Members considered themselves more intellectual than those of the older Philadelphia Club. Hidden City Philadelphia shared this member's memory: "At the Rittenhouse Club, one would find Latin commentary scribbled in the margins of the library's books. At the Philadelphia Club, the members would be most concerned with the latest racing news from Saratoga."

The **11 Barnes & Noble** bookstore is built on what was Dr. John V. Shoemaker's mansion. Shoemaker was a physician who was the National Guard's Surgeon General and Philadelphia's chief health authority.

The **12 Sarah Drexel Fell–Van Rensselaer House,** now a retail store, was completed in 1901 with a Tiffany glass dome and a ceiling covered in portraits of Italian doges.

This tour ends here, a few blocks from its beginning.

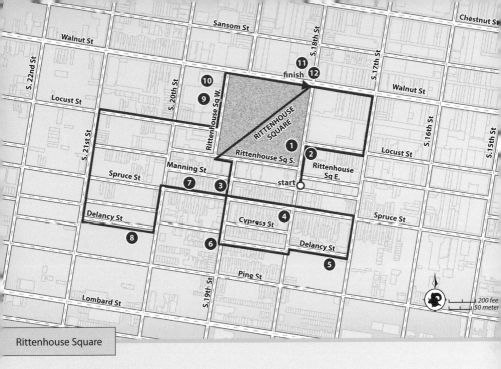

Points of Interest

1. **Rittenhouse Square** S. 18th and Walnut Sts., 267-586-5675, friendsofrittenhouse.org

2. **Curtis Institute of Music** 1726 Locust St., 215-893-5252, curtis.edu

3. **Metropolitan Bakery** 262 S. 19th St., 215-545-6655, metropolitanbakery.com

4. **Temple Beth Zion–Beth Israel Synagogue** 1800–1804 Spruce St.

5. **Plays and Players** 1714 Delancey Place, 215-735-0630, playsandplayers.org

6. **Horace Jayne House** 320 S. 19th St.

7. **Rafsnyder-Welsh House** 1923 Spruce St.

8. **Rosenbach Museum and Library** 2008–2010 Delancey Place, 215-732-1600, rosenbach.org

9. **The Rittenhouse** 201 W. Rittenhouse Square, 215-546-9000, rittenhousehotel.com

10. **Church of the Holy Trinity** 1904 Walnut St., 215-567-1267, htrit.org

11. **Barnes & Noble** 1805 Walnut St., 215-665-0716, stores.barnesandnoble.com/store/2850

12. **Sarah Drexel Fell–Van Rensselaer House** 1801 Walnut St.

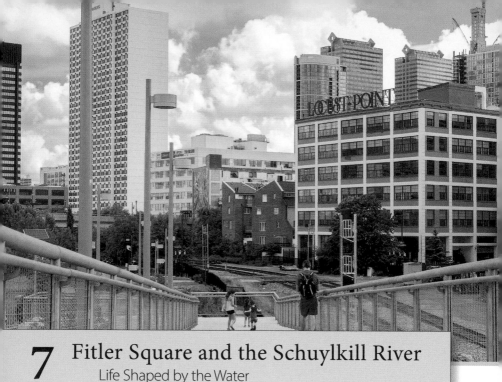

7 Fitler Square and the Schuylkill River
Life Shaped by the Water

Above: Schuylkill River Park features a waterside trail.

BOUNDARIES: Lombard St., Chestnut St., S. 22nd St., Schuylkill River
DISTANCE: 1.3 miles
DIFFICULTY: Easy
PARKING: There are no paid parking lots here; the only options are metered street parking or limited but free 2-hour street spots.
PUBLIC TRANSIT: If you're coming into the city by rail—including SEPTA and Amtrak—it's easy to exit at 30th Station and cross the Schuylkill River at South Street. By bus, the 40 or 42 will drop you a few blocks from your starting point.

The Schuylkill River wharves made Fitler Square an industrial hub in the first half of the 1800s, with coal pouring in from northern Pennsylvania's mines. Irish immigrants who worked on the water and in nearby manufacturing plants lived here.

As ships grew, business moved to the deeper and wider Delaware River. The neighborhood's fortunes declined. Urban affairs expert Jeanne Lowe described 1950s Fitler Square as a "muddle inhabited by drunks and empty bottles."

Today this neighborhood's homes, dating from the mid-19th to the 20th century, are in high demand. While real estate here costs less than properties in nearby Rittenhouse Square, it's not far off. Some people have dubbed the area between the two parks Rit-Fit or Fittenhouse Square.

Walk Description

Start at ❶ **The Philadelphia School,** at Lombard and South 25th Streets. This private institution, where tuition ranges from $27,000 to $30,500, has creatively adapted existing buildings for modern uses. Part of the main school, established in 1976, was the Philadelphia-based New York Pie Baking Company. Founder William "The Pie Man" Thompson tried to convince the public that his factory-made pies—made with pure ingredients in sterile conditions—were nutritious.

The school converted an asphalt-covered, fenced-in parking lot into a playground with green learning space. A former railroad company building became an early-childhood development center.

Walk north on South 25th Street. At Pine Street, turn right. Joseph Horn lived in the mansion at 2410 Pine Street. He and partner Frank Hardart opened their eponymous Automat chain together in 1888.

Automats operated on the same principle as vending machines. Customers viewed prepared foods behind windows, then inserted coins to lift the glass. An employee then put a fresh offering in the empty space. The country's first Automat, on nearby Chestnut Street, still has "Horn & Hardart" engraved above the doors. In 1922, a company ad boasted that one out of every 16 Philadelphians enjoyed a daily meal at an Automat.

Continue to ❷ **Fitler Square,** at 24th and Pine Streets, a half-acre park named for former Mayor Edwin Fitler, who owned a rope factory and supported the Union in the Civil War by providing uniforms for employees who served. At its center is a working Victorian-era fountain. Its three sculptures—*Fitler Square Ram, Grizzly,* and *Family of Turtles*—are self-explanatory.

Exit the square, continuing on Pine Street.

At South 22nd Street, turn left. The ❸ **Neill and Mauran Houses**—two residences under one roof—blend Colonial, Queen Anne, and medieval elements. Architect Wilson Eyre, founder of *House and Garden*, designed this structure in 1890. Note the asymmetric windows and the large doors with tiny mail slots. Eyre appears later in this walk.

Continue to ❹ **Trinity Memorial Church**, completed in the 1880s. The church's website notes, "hordes of neighbors regard it as 'their church' but do not attend—some of them regard it as such even though they are Jewish." One neighbor told a local newspaper in the 1990s, "Trinity is the glue that holds the neighborhood together."

Continue to Chandler Place (251 S. 22nd St.), built in 1904 for the bishop of Pennsylvania's Episcopal Church by Theophilus Chandler, founder of the University of Pennsylvania's Architecture Department. The building became condos in 1980. In 2021, a two-story, 1600-square-foot unit was for sale for $775,000.

The Tudor-style homes of ❺ **English Village**, at South 22nd Street and St. James Place, were built in the 1920s around a leafy pedestrian courtyard. The homes originally sold for $27,000–$30,000 and are now in the $1 million range.

Continue on South 22nd Street, crossing Walnut Street. Dr. James Hutchinson, whose grandfather founded the Philadelphia College of Physicians, lived at 133 South 22nd Street. The elder Hutchinson carried a dispatch from Benjamin Franklin in France to the Continental Congress. He became one of the Continental Army's senior surgeons, inoculating more than 3,000 soldiers against smallpox at Valley Forge. He died treating patients during the 1793 Yellow Fever epidemic.

Prominent lawyer and civic leader John Christian Bullitt lived at 125 South 22nd Street. Bullitt, whose statue stands on City Hall's north side, drafted the Philadelphia City Charter in the 1870s.

Pass Albert M. Greenfield Public School (2200 Chestnut St.). Through born in Ukraine, Greenfield got the nickname "Mr. Philadelphia" for generosity with his time and money.

At Chestnut Street, turn right. ❻ **Church of the New Jerusalem** is a Swedenborgian Church, built in 1881.

Next door, the ❼ **First Unitarian Church of Philadelphia** was designed by Frank Furness; his father, Reverend William Henry Furness, was the church leader. Reverend Furness set the church's social justice path, arguing for an end to slavery and supporting the Underground Railroad decades before the Civil War.

Continue to Van Pelt Street and turn left. The ❽ **Lutheran Church of the Holy Communion** was built for a Protestant congregation. The Lutherans came in the early 1900s, bringing their own pulpit, baptismal font, organ panel, and altar.

The nonprofit De la Salle in Towne (25 Van Pelt St.) helps boys and young men using the trauma-informed care approach. This space has historically housed charitable entities, beginning with the Evening Home for Boys, which helped homeless and uneducated boys and young men by providing food, study, fun, and guidance.

At the dead end, look right to see *Mapping Freire,* a mosaic of 6,000 photographs, mostly taken by students from Freire Charter School. The school is named for Paulo Freire, a Brazilian educator who viewed students as both teachers and learners.

Turn left on Ludlow Street. At South 22nd Street, turn left again. **❾ Mütter Museum of the College of Physicians of Philadelphia** holds a collection of medical curiosities, antique medical equipment, and many pickled things in jars. Exhibits include a tumor removed from President Grover Cleveland, the liver of conjoined twins Chang and Eng, slides of Einstein's brain, and tissue from John Wilkes Booth's thorax. A glass case holds the 8-foot-long colon removed from a man who had complained of constipation for most of his life.

To the right of the entrance is the Benjamin Rush Medicinal Plant Garden. Rush—a signer of the Declaration of Independence and founding member of the College of Physicians—wanted a garden where colleagues could replenish their supplies. The four beds of plantings contain more than 60 medicinal plants, including spiderwort, used in laxatives.

With your back to the garden, look across South 22nd Street. At right is Sidney Hillman Apartments, or Sidneyville, subsidized senior housing built in 1969 by the Philadelphia Men's Garment Workers Union and named for labor leader/FDR confidante Sidney Hillman.

At left is Wilson Eyre Condominiums, named for the architect. Built in the 1880s for a University of Pennsylvania literary society, the first floor was a social club with living space above. The exterior is adorned with what appears to be screaming or smirking doll heads. One website said the babies are singing.

Continue on South 22nd Street. At Chestnut Street, turn right. The Coronado (2201 Chestnut St.), now condominiums, was built in 1910. Pass Greenfield School. At South 23rd Street, turn right.

The ❿ **23rd Street Armory**, a granite fortress in the middle of the city, is the home of the First Troop, Philadelphia City Cavalry, which is now part of the Pennsylvania National Guard. The unit, formed in 1774, served as George Washington's personal bodyguards during the Revolutionary War while also fighting by his side.

At Market Street, turn left. Continue to the Schuylkill River. Take the pedestrian ramp next to the eagle statue at left to reach the trail below.

At the bottom of the ramp, turn left and pass under the Walnut Street bridge. Bear right around a center planting, then keep right to traverse the Schuylkill Banks Boardwalk.

Before the South Street Bridge, exit via the ramp at left. *Convergence* (South St. and Schuylkill Banks) is composed of differently colored crisscrossing shapes meant to mirror the area's transportation networks.

Exit onto South Street opposite CHOP's Roberts Pediatric Research Center. Turn left. The single human figure in *Welcome to the Neighborhood* (S. 27th and South Sts.) is artist David Guinn.

Turn left onto Taney Street, with the Philadelphia School at right. At Naudain Street, turn right. These final parts of the walk wander Fitler's lovely residential streets. At South 25th Street, turn left. At Lombard Street, turn right. At South 24th Street, turn left. At Waverly Street, turn right. When you reach South 23rd Street, turn left, passing Fitler Square on the left.

At Delancey Place, turn left and walk to the final stop, **11** **Schuylkill River Park,** which includes two dog runs, a community garden, and the perfect place to sit after a long walk.

The beginnings of the Rittenhouse Square (page 33) and West Philadelphia II (page 171) tours are nearby.

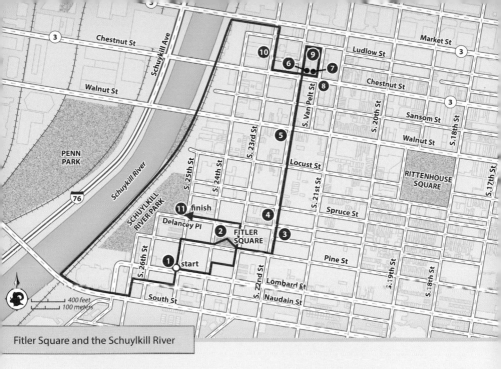

Fitler Square and the Schuylkill River

Points of Interest

1 The Philadelphia School 2503 Lombard St., 215-545-5323, tpschool.org

2 Fitler Square 23rd and Pine Sts., fitlersquare.org

3 Neill and Mauran Houses 315–17 S. 22nd St.

4 Trinity Memorial Church 2212 Spruce St., 215-732-2515, trinityphiladelphia.org

5 English Village S. 22nd St. and St. James Place

6 Church of the New Jerusalem 2129 Chestnut St.

7 First Unitarian Church of Philadelphia 2125 Chestnut St., 215-563-3980, philauu.org

8 Lutheran Church of the Holy Communion 2110 Chestnut St., 215-567-3668, lc-hc.org

9 Mütter Museum of the College of Physicians of Philadelphia 19 S. 22nd St., 215-563-3737, muttermuseum.org

10 23rd Street Armory 22 S. 23rd St., 215-564-1488, 23rdstreetarmory.org

11 Schuylkill River Park 300 S. 25th St., fsrp.org

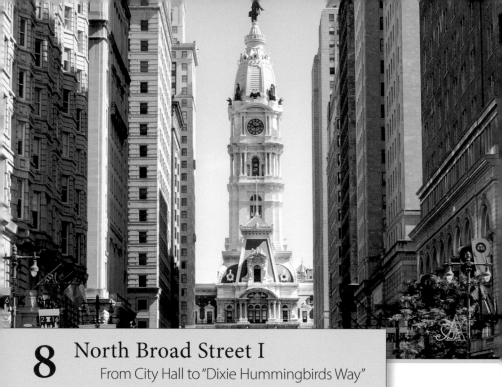

8 North Broad Street I
From City Hall to "Dixie Hummingbirds Way"

Above: Philadelphia's ornate City Hall is topped with a statue of founder William Penn.

BOUNDARIES: Broad St., John F. Kennedy Blvd., Poplar St.
DISTANCE: 1.3 miles
DIFFICULTY: Easy
PARKING: Public parking is limited, and private parking can be costly.
PUBLIC TRANSIT: Take SEPTA to the City Hall station via the Broad Street line or one of the numerous buses that circle the plaza.

At 12 miles long, Broad Street is the country's longest straight city street. The northern section developed more slowly than its southern stretch, despite attempts by well-known residents—including department store magnate Ellis Gimbel and actor Edwin Forrest—to make it a Millionaire's Row.

Walk Description

Begin on the north side of ❶ **City Hall,** North Broad Street and John F. Kennedy Boulevard, to see two statues of men atop horses. At right is General John Fulton Reynolds, a decorated soldier killed at the Battle of Gettysburg. This was the city's first public monument to a Civil War soldier and its first equestrian statue.

At left is Civil War General George McClellan, the "Hero of Antietam." McClellan helped the army develop its standard-issue saddle, which is why people were angry that this statue shows a horse with an ill-fitting bridle.

Walk to the corner of North 15th Street and John F. Kennedy Boulevard, following the cross-walks across JFK to the ❷ **Municipal Services Building** and its art-filled plaza.

Government of the People, a 30-foot-tall totem pole–like sculpture, was commissioned for the bicentennial, only for critics to say it looked like a pile of crushed people. The Association for Public Art disagreed, writing, "As a symbol of democracy, the sculpture suggests a process of continual struggle, mutual support and dedication, and eventual triumph."

Circle the plaza to see the game pieces—from Monopoly, Parcheesi, dominoes, chess, and checkers—that make up *Your Move.* An artist involved in the work said the sculptures juxtapose carefree childhood memories with adult responsibilities, which city workers undoubtedly appreciate Mondays at 8 a.m.

Leave the plaza via the front steps. Turn left. Walk to North Broad Street. Turn left again. *Benjamin Franklin, Craftsman,* at North Broad Street and John F. Kennedy Boulevard, was commissioned by the nearby Masonic temple. Fans say this sculpture, depicting Franklin as a young man instead of full bellied and balding, is a welcome change. Others complain the proportions seem uneven.

The ❸ **Masonic Temple** is the headquarters of the Grand Lodge of Pennsylvania, Free and Accepted Masons. Freemasonry is the world's oldest continuously existing fraternal organization. Many Founding Fathers, including George Washington, were Freemasons.

The cathedral–like building was completed in 1873, but the elaborate interior—which includes seven lodge rooms, each designed in a different period style—took another 20 years to finish. Each room has one intentional flaw to signify man's imperfection. Washington's Masonic apron, embroidered by the Marquis de Lafayette's wife, is displayed in the library. In 1902, the Masonic Temple became one of the city's first fully electrified buildings.

The neighboring ❹ **Arch Street United Methodist Church** was built in 1870 atop a coal yard. The Gothic marble structure has always housed a forward-thinking congregation. Church leader Matthew Simpson delivered the eulogy at President Abraham Lincoln's funeral. The church remains socially active and has a welcoming congregation.

Continue north. ❺ **Pennsylvania Academy of the Fine Arts** is headquartered in an 1806 building that combines Second Empire, creative Renaissance, and elegant Gothic architectural styles. Above the door is a headless statue of Ceres, Greek goddess of the harvest.

Continue to *Paint Torch*, which stands 51 feet high and leans at a 60-degree angle. Artist Claes Oldenburg also created the *Clothespin* sculpture near City Hall. A 2015 *Philadelphia* article wondered if Philadelphia was the only city to "get suckered in" by Oldenburg, noting "Right now, he's likely over in Stockholm rubbing his palms together and wondering what new eyesore he can pawn off on our oh-so-gullible citizenry. We really have got to learn to say no to giant household items."

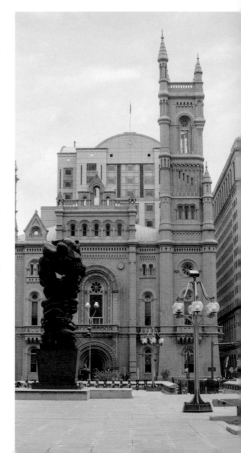

The Masonic Temple with Government of the People in the foreground

Continue north. *Declaration* (150 N. Broad St.) is one of the city's newest and largest murals. It features the face of a woman of color with the antislavery section of the Declaration of Independence, removed before ratification, superimposed on her face. The message? Despite the document's lofty language, rights were never meant to be granted equally.

❻ *How to Turn Anything into Something Else* is a fantastical mural designed by students challenged to consider obstacles as opportunity. A lemon becomes a bird, a boat transforms into a whale. The young artists say the girl at top is the strongest woman in the world.

❼ *Independence Starts Here* is on the side of Hahnemann University Hospital, which closed in 2019. The fate of the building and the mural are unknown. Note the American Sign Language finger alphabet spelling out the word *independence*. Students from the Pennsylvania School for the Deaf posed for the artist.

Stop at Vine Street. Turn around to see **8** *The Evolving Face of Nursing*, which encourages viewers to see nurses in different ways. Artist Meg Saligman interviewed more than 100 nurses and included their faces and words in the mural. It's the first city mural to use LED lighting technology.

Roman Catholic High School (301 N. Broad St.) dates to 1890 and was the country's first school to offer a free parochial education. The Packard Motor Corporation Building (317–32 N. Broad St.) originally housed a showroom and offices for the Packard company. It is now condos. Built in 1911, the seven-story structure was one of the country's first made using reinforced concrete in a steel frame.

This stretch was once known as Automobile Row. A 1910 photo shows multiple auto dealerships, including Ford, Oldsmobile, Hudson, and Buick.

The parking garage across the street replaced the Broadwood Hotel, which in the 1920s became the home court of the South Philadelphia Hebrew Association (SPHAs), putting an end to the team nickname "the Wandering Jews."

Continue north. **9** **The Inquirer Building,** the 18-story white building at Broad and Callowhill Streets, once housed the city's two daily newspapers, *The Philadelphia Inquirer* and *The Philadelphia Daily News*. Friends—and enemies—called the building "The Tower of Truth."

In a city of few skyscrapers, this building, with its gold dome and four-faced clock that is visible for miles, had a major impact when it was completed in 1924. As newspapers declined, the media entities moved to a smaller location. The building was sold in 2011.

Next door, The School District of Philadelphia's headquarters (444 N. Broad St.) serves more than 200,000 students. During the 1950s Red Scare, veteran teacher Herman Beilan refused to answer questions about his Communist party affiliations and was fired for "incompetency." Beilan sued, saying he had been denied due process. The U.S Supreme Court sided with the District in a 5–4 decision because by refusing to respond to his superiors, "Beilan showed himself to be insubordinate and lacking in frankness, which gave the Board grounds to fire him," oyez.org reports.

Continue to Spring Garden Street. Another Saligman mural, **10** *Common Threads,* on the right, features students from two nearby high schools and dolls that belonged to the artist's grandmother.

Farther north, on the left, is *All Join Hands: Visions of Peace* (550 N. Broad St.). The design was inspired by a yearlong, citywide antiviolence initiative.

In the 1800s, this intersection was an industrial hub, part of the sprawling 17-acre Baldwin Locomotive Works. Company founder Matthias Baldwin designed *Old Ironsides,* one of the country's first successful locomotives. Assembling the train was such an involved process that, when it was finished, Baldwin declared, "This is the last locomotive that we'll ever build." Instead, the company became the world's largest locomotive maker. At its peak, the company was churning out 2,500 locomotives annually and shipping them as far as Siberia.

⓫ **Congregation Rodeph Shalom** is the oldest Ashkenazi Jewish congregation in the Western Hemisphere, founded in 1795 by worshippers from Germany, Holland, and Poland. Published in 1975, *The History of the Jews of Philadelphia from Colonial Times Until the Age of Jackson* notes that the congregation offered free membership to the poor and rabbis gave money to those in need, with the expectation the recipients would attend weekly services. The Moorish synagogue contains the Philadelphia Museum of Jewish Art and the Obermayer Collection of Jewish Ritual Art.

Continue on North Broad Street, passing Old Zion Lutheran Church (628 N. Broad St.), which has a congregation dating to 1752. German remains one of the church's official languages. "Not even the two World Wars were enough to muzzle our preachers," the church website says.

Continue north. ⓬ **Clementine's Stable Café** occupies a 19th-century horse stable. Pass Wallace Street, also called Samuel Staten Sr. Drive in remembrance of a longtime leader of the Laborers' Union who died in 2016. The Studebaker building (667 N. Broad St.) is a mixed-use commercial building originally built as a car showroom.

The ⓭ **Divine Lorraine Hotel** is named for charismatic Father Major Jealous Divine. His church, Universal Peace Mission Movement, purchased the Lorraine Hotel in 1948. The Gilded Age beauty, built in 1894, became the country's first fully racially integrated hotel. Visitors had to follow church rules, which included no smoking, drinking, or profanity. Women and men had rooms on separate floors, and modesty—in part meaning women had to wear skirts—was enforced.

Pass the Salvation Army headquarters (701 N. Broad St.), then turn to see the mural on its

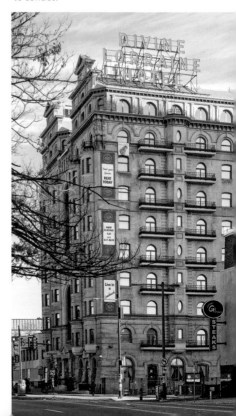

The Divine Lorraine Hotel, abandoned and empty for decades, is currently being converted to condos.

north wall featuring a smiling bell ringer. The organization's annual red kettle campaign began in San Francisco in 1891 when an organization member set a kettle near the Oakland Ferry Landing and asked passersby to "Keep the pot boiling" with a monetary donation. In 2019, the bell ringers collected $126 million.

Opposite is the **⓮ Greater Exodus Baptist Church**, built in 1877 for a Presbyterian congregation, and a Baptist ministry since the 1970s. The church was failing when, in 1982, former Philadelphia Eagle Herbert H. Lusk II became minister. Under Lusk, the church has thrived, with more than 2,000 members. The historic building features a vestibule mural depicting the history of African American Baptists.

Continue on Broad Street and pass Parrish Street. The **⓯ Philadelphia Metropolitan Opera House** was built by Oscar Hammerstein, grandfather of the famous lyricist, as competition for the popular Academy of Music on South Broad Street. Local newspapers predicted wealthy locals would never travel north to see a show. The rivalry was tested on opening night in 1908, when The Met offered a production of *Carmen* with a 700-member cast and the Academy presented beloved opera singer Enrico Caruso. Both venues sold out. According to reports, the Academy audience listened to Caruso until intermission, then headed uptown to watch the second half of *Carmen*.

The Met closed after two sold-out seasons. It reopened as an entertainment venue in 2018 after a two-year, $56-million renovation. Bob Dylan performed the inaugural concert.

This stretch of North Broad Street is also known as Dixie Hummingbirds Way in honor of the Grammy-winning gospel quartet. In 1983, the band wrote the song "Moses is Going to Take Us to the Promised Land" to celebrate the Philadelphia 76ers basketball team and star player Moses Malone as the team faced the Los Angeles Lakers in the NBA championship. The 76ers won the series four games to none.

This walk ends here. The second North Broad Street walk (page 53) begins in the 1200 block of North Broad Street.

Points of Interest

1 **City Hall** 1401 John F. Kennedy Blvd., 215-686-1776, phila.gov

2 **Municipal Services Building** 1401 John F. Kennedy Blvd., 215-686-8686, phila.gov

3 **Masonic Temple** 1 N. Broad St., 215-988-1900, pamasonictemple.org

4 **Arch Street United Methodist Church** 55 N. Broad St., archstreetumc.org

(continued on next page)

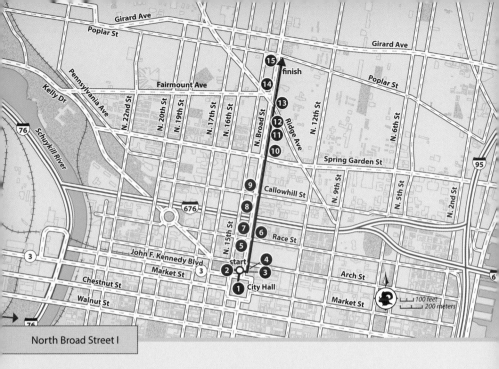

(continued from previous page)

5 **Pennsylvania Academy of the Fine Arts** 118–128 N. Broad St., 215-972-7600, pafa.org

6 *How to Turn Anything into Something Else* 207 N. Broad St., Mural Arts Philadelphia, 215-685-0750, muralarts.org

7 *Independence Starts Here* 216 N. Broad St., Mural Arts Philadelphia, 215-685-0750, muralarts.org

8 *The Evolving Face of Nursing* N. Broad and Vine Sts., Mural Arts Philadelphia, 215-685-0750, muralarts.org

9 **The Inquirer Building** 400 N. Broad St.

10 *Common Threads* N. Broad and Spring Garden Sts., Mural Arts Philadelphia, 215-685-0750, muralarts.org

11 **Congregation Rodeph Shalom** 615 N. Broad St., 215-627-6747, rodephshalom.org

12 **Clementine's Stable Café** 631 N. Broad St., 215-454–6530, clementinescafe.com

13 **Divine Lorraine Hotel** 699 N. Broad St., thedivinelorrainehotel.com

14 **Greater Exodus Baptist Church** 704 N. Broad St., 215-235-1394, gebch.com

15 **Philadelphia Metropolitan Opera House** 858 N. Broad St.

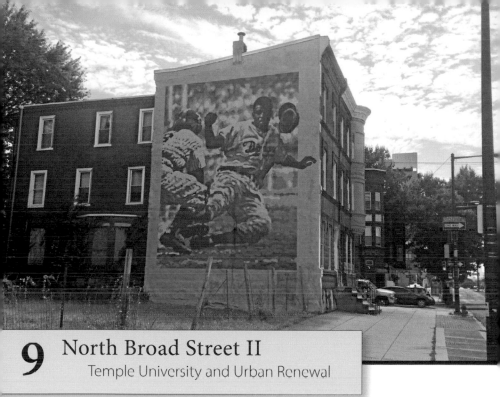

9 North Broad Street II
Temple University and Urban Renewal

Above: Jackie Robinson successfully slides into home in this mural.

BOUNDARIES: Girard Ave., Glenwood Ave., N. Broad St.
DISTANCE: 1.8 miles
DIFFICULTY: Easy
PARKING: There are two public parking garages on the Temple University campus.
PUBLIC TRANSIT: SEPTA's Broad Street Line stops near Temple University at N. 10th and Berks Sts. Bus stops within 0.5 mile include the C bus, 3, and 23.

Broad Street is the longest straight urban road in America, part of the original city plan. There is no 14th Street in the street grid between the Delaware and the Schuylkill Rivers; Broad Street has taken its place. Someone who gives directions to a location on 14th Street is a prankster. This stretch of Broad has been heavily influenced by ever-expanding Temple University.

Walk Description

Start at North Broad Street and Girard Avenue. *North Philadelphia Heroes* (1214 N. Broad St.) honors seven locals, including Dr. Ethel Allen, the city's first African American councilwoman and physician, and Lillia "Mom" Crippen, whose 1999 obituary called her "a one-woman social-service agency." Crippen had a hand in the raising of as many as 40 children, many of them handicapped and unwanted. In 1988, she told the *Philadelphia Inquirer,* "All you have to do is say you don't want them and I'll take them."

Continue north. *The Legendary Blue Horizon* (1314 N. Broad St.) remembers the 1,500-seat boxing venue that closed in 2010. Made up of three circa-19th-century houses, the Horizon was a sporting hot spot in the 1960s. Featured fighters include Muhammad Ali, Joe Frazier, Larry "The Easton Assassin" Holmes, and George Foreman.

Walk north. The Italianate building housing ❶ **New Freedom Theatre** was actor Edwin Forrest's home until he died in 1872. Philadelphia-born Forrest was a teenager when he took part in a laughing gas experiment and delivered a Shakespearean soliloquy under its influence. Someone who witnessed the performance introduced Forrest to a local acting troop, thus launching his career. In May 1849, Forrest's fans clashed with supporters of rival actor William Macready in New York's Astor Place Riot, killing at least 22 people. New Freedom, Pennsylvania's oldest African American theater company, moved into the building in 1968.

The building at 1430 N. Broad St. was erected in the 1890s for Charles Ellis, who made his fortune operating a horse-drawn trolley company. Ellis died in 1909. His $4 million estate established the Charles E. Ellis College for Fatherless Girls. The college closed in 1977, but the trust fund continues to help young women, awarding more than $1 million in education grants annually.

The Beaux Arts Alfred E. Burk House (1500 N. Broad St.) dates to 1909. Historian and author Robert Morris Skaler called it "the last great mansion built on North Broad Street." Burk and his brothers owned a leather-goods factory mentioned in the Northern Liberties walk.

❷ **Sullivan Progress Plaza,** the country's oldest African American–developed and –owned shopping center, exists thanks to Baptist minister Leon Sullivan. The so-called "Lion of Zion" led efforts in the 1960s to develop this shopping plaza for this underserved African American neighborhood. Sullivan, awarded the Presidential Medal of Freedom in 1999, is on the center panel of a mural decorating the center.

Cross Oxford Street. The main campus of Temple University, a state-related institution, sprawls across 105 acres. About 28,000 undergraduate and 10,000 graduate students are currently enrolled.

Rock Hall (1715 N. Broad St.) was built for the Reform Congregation Keneseth Israel and now houses Temple's music school. Its name does not refer to rock and roll but to Dr. Milton Rock, who funded its renovation. The James E. Beasley School of Law (1719 N. Broad St.) is named for the flamboyant trial lawyer whose biography is *Courtroom Cowboy*.

Cecil B. Moore Avenue honors the lawyer and civil rights activist who worked with Martin Luther King Jr. and Malcolm X. Moore also served on the Philadelphia City Council and was president of the Philadelphia chapter of the NAACP. A 1987 *The Philadelphia Inquirer* article described him as a "loud, cigar-chomping man who demanded—and got— respect."

Temple University's Liacouras Center (1776 N. Broad St.) honors Peter J. Liacouras, university president from 1981 to 2000. Liacouras is credited with transforming Temple from a "commuter school on North Broad Street to . . . a world-class institution," his 2016 obituary noted. He promoted the university with a marketing campaign featuring famous alums saying, "We could have gone anywhere. We chose Temple."

Continue past Conwell Hall, built in 1929 and named for university founder Russell Conwell. The ❸ **Temple Performing Arts Center** occupies the former Grace Baptist Church, which Conwell once led. In 1882, a young man in Conwell's congregation asked the minister to tutor him. Soon Conwell was teaching a group of men in the evenings. They were dubbed the Night Owls, inadvertently naming Temple's future sports teams. The Temple College charter was issued in 1888 with Conwell as its president.

A popular speaker, Conwell gave his "Acres of Diamonds" lecture more than 6,000 times between 1869 and 1925. The speech, later a book, proposed that people don't need to travel far to find success because all they need is within their home community. The title comes from an anecdote about a man who sold his property to search for riches, only to have the property's new owner discover a diamond mine.

The center also has a Chapel of the Four Chaplains, which honors four Army chaplains from different religious orders who, when the SS *Dorchester* was sinking after being struck by a U-boat torpedo in February 1945, treated the wounded, calmed the panicked, and gave up their own life jackets and lives.

Legend says the men linked arms on the ship's deck and sang and prayed as the boat sank. One witness said, "It was the finest thing I have seen or hope to see this side of heaven." Only 230 men of the 904 aboard survived. In 1988, Congress unanimously voted to establish February 3 as Four Chaplains Day.

Continue on North Broad Street, crossing Berks Street. Across the road, the low stone wall is a remnant of Monument Cemetery, a sprawling Victorian garden–style resting place modeled after Paris's Père Lachaise. In the 1950s, more than 20,000 bodies were dug up and moved so Temple University could build sports fields and parking lots. Many cemetery headstones were used to construct the base of the Betsy Ross Bridge. Luke Barley wrote on citylab.com that "at low tide, some of the headstones are still visible, no longer a testament to a person beneath, but to the uniquely American habit of turning anything, paradise or cemetery, into a parking lot."

Continue on North Broad Street. The 1895 residence of real estate developer John Stafford (2000 N. Broad St.) is the Alpha Epsilon Pi fraternity house. A 2009 article in the *Temple News* detailed paranormal activity there, including doors opening and closing, items disappearing, and footsteps climbing the stairs.

The mural at North Broad and Diamond Streets depicts Grover Washington Jr., the American jazz/funk/soul saxophonist who is often credited—or blamed—with creating the smooth jazz genre. ❹ **Berean Presbyterian Church** was founded by Pastor Matthew Anderson in 1880. Anderson used his platform to improve the lives of African Americans by encouraging home ownership—he established a loan company to finance purchases—and opening a trade school. His wife, Caroline Still, the daughter of an Underground Railroad conductor and one of the nation's first African American female doctors, supported his work.

❺ **Uptown Theater** was a major venue on the so-called chitlin circuit between 1951 and 1978, welcoming comedians such as Redd Foxx and Flip Wilson. Still a community gathering point, residents congregated outside after singer Michael Jackson's death in 2009.

WDAS/WHAT AM radio DJ Georgie Woods promoted shows here. Known on the airwaves as "the guy with the goods," Woods used the AM radio airwaves to promote the civil rights movement. In 1963, he helped charter 21 buses to take people to the March on Washington.

Woods was so influential that when race riots broke out blocks from the theater in 1964, police asked him to calm the crowds, which disbanded at his request. The NAACP later honored Woods. A nearby sign designates this stretch as Georgie Woods Boulevard.

Continue north. Dropsie College for Hebrew and Cognate Learning (2331 N. Broad St.) closed in 1986. Faculty members included Benzion Netanyahu, whose son Benjamin would become Israeli prime minister.

The Philadelphia and Reading Railroad's former North Broad Street Station (2601 N. Broad St.) was built in the 1920s and closed in the 1960s because of dwindling ridership. It's now low-income housing.

The gray warehouse across the street (2622 N. Broad St.) was the Baker Bowl, the Philadelphia Phillies' home field. Officially called National League Park, the stadium cost $80,000 to build in 1887 and comfortably sat 12,000. Here, Pittsburgh's Honus Wagner slammed his 3,000th career

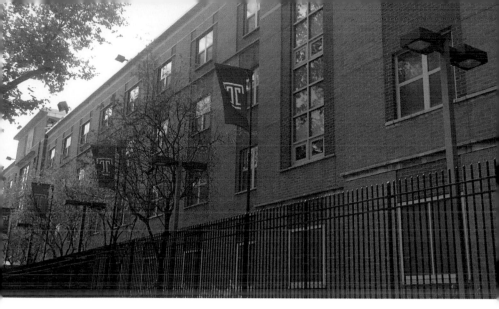

Temple University's continued growth means ongoing change on North Broad Street.

hit in June 1914, President Woodrow Wilson became the first president to attend the World Series, and Babe Ruth played his final major league game.

A colorful mural on the building at North Broad Street and Lehigh Avenue reads *SHINE*. Remember that.

The 10 story former Ford Motor Company Assembly Plant (2700 N. Broad St.), now empty, produced about 150 cars each day from 1910 to 1926. After World War I, the company moved to the suburbs.

Turn around to read *RISE* on the opposite side of the building at North Broad Street and Lehigh Avenue.

Continue on North Broad Street to ❻ *Tribute to Jackie Robinson.* This 30-foot-tall mural honors the athlete who desegregated Major League Baseball in 1947. Artist David McShane used black and white paint as a reminder of Robinson's struggles. The image, a compilation of two photos, shows Robinson, a Brooklyn Dodger, stealing home in the 1955 World Series against the New York Yankees. The opposing catcher, No. 8, is Yogi Berra. The umpire called Robinson safe, although video footage indicates otherwise. Berra always insisted Robinson was out.

Cross Glenwood Avenue, passing the North Philadelphia Station, opened in the 1870s to serve the city's subway line and Amtrak.

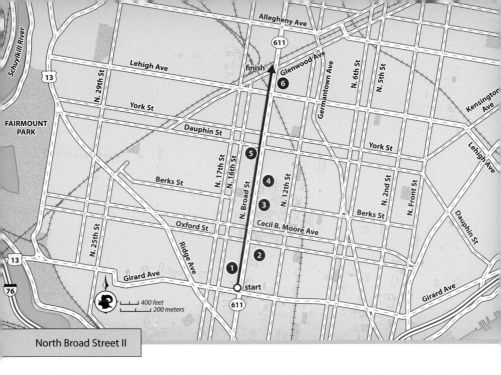

The final stop is one block north. The former furniture store with yellow-and-red signage (2917 N. Broad St.) was boxer Joe Frazier's gym. The Olympic gold medalist and World Heavyweight Champion, perhaps best remembered for beating Muhammad Ali in 1971's Fight of the Century, trained fighters here for 25 years. His name is still engraved above the front door.

Points of Interest

1. **New Freedom Theatre** 1346 N. Broad St., 888-802-8998, freedomtheatre.org
2. **Sullivan Progress Plaza** 1501 N. Broad St., 215-232-7070, progressplaza.com
3. **Temple Performing Arts Center** 1837 N. Broad St., 215-204-9860, templeperformingartscenter.org
4. **Berean Presbyterian Church** 2101 N. Broad St., bereanpresbyterian.org
5. **Uptown Theater (now closed)** 2240–2248 N. Broad St.
6. *Tribute to Jackie Robinson* 2803 N. Broad St., Mural Arts Philadelphia, 215-685-0750, muralarts.org

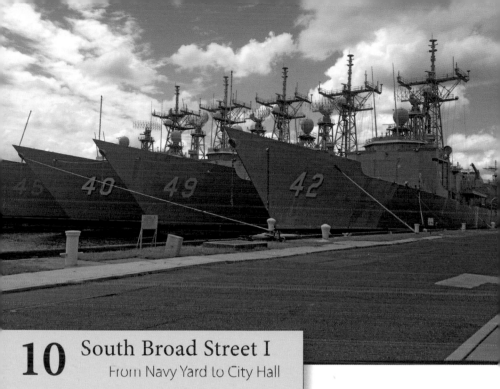

10 South Broad Street I
From Navy Yard to City Hall

BOUNDARIES: S. Broad St., Market St., Constitution Ave.
DISTANCE: 3.9 miles; if you loop through the Navy Yard, add another 1.4 miles
DIFFICULTY: Moderate
PARKING: Metered street parking is available once the walk passes the stadium area. The sporting complexes have multiple pay lots.
PUBLIC TRANSIT: SEPTA's Broad Street line stops at AT&T station, near the stadiums, about 0.2 mile away. The Navy Yard also offers a free shuttle between Center City and the Navy Yard. The stop is at N. 10th St. between Market and Filbert Sts. The schedule is available online.

Broad Street is where the city celebrates: where mummers have paraded for a century (for more on the Mummers Parade, see Walk 24, page 158), where residents gathered to mark the end of World Wars I and II, and where sports teams have victory parades.

Walk Description

Begin at the ❶ **Philadelphia Navy Yard**, the first Unites States Navy shipyard. The current facilities were built in the 1870s. During World War II, the yard employed more than 40,000 people who built 53 ships, including the USS *New Jersey*. Workers repaired almost 600 war-damaged crafts, and scientists developed the liquid thermal diffusion technique that made the Manhattan Project possible.

Most Navy programs here closed in the 1990s. City government converted the area into a thriving business hub, with more than 150 companies—including pharmaceutical giant GlaxoSmithKline and retailer Urban Outfitters—employing more than 13,500 people. (The Navy Yard's management has designed a self-guided, 2-mile walking tour of the 1,200-acre property that's available at navyyard.org.)

Begin walking north on South Broad Street. On the right past I-95 is the ❷ **South Philadelphia Sports Complex.** This is where the city's professional sporting teams play—Citizens Bank Park for baseball's Phillies; the Wells Fargo Center for hockey's Flyers and basketball's 76ers; and Lincoln Financial Field for football's Eagles.

In 2016, Hillary Clinton became the first female presidential nominee from a major party when she accepted the Democratic Party's nomination at the Wells Fargo Center, which opened in 1996. The other two facilities opened in the early 2000s. Two additional key parts of the complex are XFinity Live! (1100 Pattinson Ave.), a retail/entertainment center, and Live! Casino and Hotel Philadelphia (900 Packer Ave.), a $700-million project completed in 2021.

Continue on South Broad Street. Cars are often parked in the middle of the street despite a law forbidding it. As a 2017 *Philadelphia Inquirer* article observed, "If you've lived in Philly longer than it takes to boil an egg, you know that the law against parking in the median of Broad Street simply vanishes between Washington and Oregon Avenue. In 1961, when Mayor Richardson Dilworth proposed stopping the practice at a South Philadelphia town hall meeting, about 2,000 angry residents howled and hurled tomatoes at him. Dilworth's lesson was internalized into the fabric of the city, and the odd custom of parking in the middle of a state highway … became a political third rail."

Continue north, passing I-76 to Marconi Plaza (2800 S. Broad St.). Guglielmo Marconi's statue was dedicated on April 25, 1980, the 106th anniversary of the Italian scientist/inventor/Nobel Prize Laureate's birth. The *Father of Modern Communications* is an unimposing figure, wearing a neat suit with his hands by his sides. Marconi's humble nature was one of his beloved traits.

Cross Oregon Avenue. The Children's House of Philadelphia (2611 S. Broad St.) was originally a church, then a restaurant. It became a school in 2018.

Continue north, passing Shunk Street, which is named for Francis Rawn Shunk, the 10th governor of Pennsylvania. Monti-Rago Funeral Home (2531–35 Broad St.) is one of about a dozen funeral homes on South Broad Street bearing an Italian surname. A 1974 *Western Folklore* article described how many Italian immigrants brought peasant customs to the US, including removing a body from a home feet first so the deceased would be unable to see the home's address and return later. Another custom was burying the dead with useful objects, including cigarettes, money, and matches. If something was forgotten, "it would often be sent in the casket of another villager who died later with hope that the two souls would meet."

At Porter Street, Bambi Cleaners (2439 S. Broad St.) has been in operation since the 1950s and has a sign with a look-alike Disney deer from days when copyright laws were more lax. Philadelphia Performing Arts Charter School (2407 S. Broad St.) holds the kindergarten and first grade classes of String Theory Schools, which equally emphasize academic and artistic excellence.

Continue north for two blocks. ❸ **South Philadelphia High School** was built in 1907 as the Southern Manual Training High School for boys, primarily Italian and Jewish immigrants. Alum Israel Goldstein graduated from the University of Pennsylvania at age 17 and went on to become a well-known rabbi and founder of Brandeis University. Other notable graduates include Chubby Checker, Eddie Fisher, Jack Klugman, and Marian Anderson. Less recognizable is Eddie "Mr. Basketball" Gottlieb. In the 1920s, Gottlieb cofounded the Philadelphia Sphas (pronounced "spas"), a basketball team named for its sponsor, South Philadelphia Hebrew Association. Most players were Jewish. For years, the team had no home court and was known as The Wandering Jews.

In 1946, Gottlieb's Philadelphia Warriors won the NBA's first championship. He later helmed the NBA's rules committee for 25 years and handled scheduling for 30 years. Basketball Hall of Famer Larry Litwack said, "Gottlieb was about as important to the game of basketball as the basketball."

The school's vibrant mural, *Parts Per Million,* highlights the school's diversity and includes 27 flags representing each language spoken by Southern students. When it was dedicated in 2019, Mural Arts Philadelphia Director Jane Golden said, "Our kids deserve to be in beautiful learning environments, and it has so much power if kids can see their thoughts and ideas on a large scale, permanently."

Continue north. The building at 2037 South Broad Street was a bank, then a fast-food restaurant, and now it's empty. On the opposite corner, Citizens Bank (2001 S. Broad St.) was built for the Philadelphia Savings Fund Society.

Continue, crossing McKean, Mifflin, Moore, and Morris Streets, each named for a former Pennsylvania governor.

At the Tasker Street intersection, Philadelphia Gas Works (1601 S. Broad St.) and Dolphin Billiards Tavern (1539 S. Broad St.) both have interesting signs.

Pennsylvania Burial Company/Baldi Funeral Home (1327–29 S. Broad St., past Reed St.) was opened in 1921 by Italian immigrant Pietro Jacovini, creator of the prepaid funeral. Jacovini was editor of the city's Italian-language newspaper and a civic leader who led the New Year's Day parade on his black stallion.

76ers: Beyond the Court, on 1203 S. Broad Street, features some of the team's biggest stars, including Allen Iverson, Charles Barkley, Julius "Dr. J" Erving, and Wilt Chamberlain. Artist Ernel Martinez took inspiration from 11-year-old Brendan Dougherty, whose mural concept won a contest. Brendan's drawing is on the lower right.

Philip's Restaurant (1145 S. Broad St.) closed in the 1990s, but the sign remains. When the restaurant opened in the 1940s, owner Philip Muzi only used his first name because the nation was at war with Italy. The building's landscape mural dates to Mural Arts Philadelphia's earliest days, when its primary goal was covering graffiti.

Cross Ellsworth Street. While the sign for the Boot & Saddle bar remains (1131 S. Broad St.), it closed in 2020. The Boot was the city's only country-Western bar for more than two decades before it was shuttered in 1995. It reopened in 2013 as a live-music venue before becoming a casualty of the COVID-19 shutdown.

At the Washington Avenue intersection, the empty plot at 1001 S. Broad Street was Citizens Volunteer Hospital, which treated wounded Union soldiers. Opened in 1863, the hospital had 400 beds but routinely treated double that number. In an odd coincidence, the hospital was within view of the station where Union soldiers boarded trains heading south.

The ❹ **Philadelphia High School for Creative and Performing Arts (CAPA)** was built in 1907 as a library, holding the tomb of the couple who built the Greek Revival building. The library closed in the 1960s, and the building suffered, at one point looking so run-down that it was used as a backdrop in 1995's *Twelve Monkeys* to show a destroyed city. CAPA moved here in 1997. (The entombed couple moved out—or were moved.) Famous alums include members of The Roots. This section of road has been renamed to honor R&B vocal group Boyz II Men, CAPA graduates whose songs include "End of the Road" and "I'll Make Love to You."

The Philadelphia Fire Department's Engine 1, Ladder 5 (711 S. Broad St.) moved to this station in 1964. In June 1973, 40 firefighters, including every member of Ladder 5, were injured and two firefighters were killed while fighting an eight-alarm fire in an ink factory on nearby Washington Avenue.

Arts Bank (601 S. Broad St.), now performance spaces, opened in 1886 as South Philadelphia National Bank. The bank printed $1.5 million between 1886 and 1935.

The 1882 Queen Anne–style home at 507 S. Broad St. belonged to J. Dundas Lippincott. The Lippincotts founded their eponymous publishing company in 1785 and sold it in 1978 to what is now HarperCollins. **5** *Theatre of Life,* one of the city's most popular murals, shows different figures representing roles people play. The hands holding marionette sticks symbolize external influences that control people. Mosaics accent the painting, giving it a 3-D effect. The mural required 400 gallons of paint, 10,000 pieces of glass, and 5,000 marbles.

The **6** **University of the Arts Lightbox Film Center** occupies what was once the Gershman Y, a cultural and community center since 1924. Its mission changed in 2018. YM&WHA—Young Men and Women's Hebrew Association—is carved on the facade.

7 **Broad Street Ministry,** founded in 2005, self-identifies as a "broad-minded Christian community that practices radical hospitality and works for a more just world through civic engagement." A former pastor called its weekly community meal "Philadelphia's most dangerous dinner party," bringing together 4,000 diners from all economic stratas.

The building at 309 S. Broad Street housed Philadelphia International Records, a Motown Records rival where songwriters/producers Kenneth Gamble and Leon Huff created "The Sound of Philadelphia." Its top-selling acts included Patti LaBelle, Teddy Pendergrass, and Lou Rawls. The label's hits include "Ain't No Stoppin' Us Now" and "TSOP (The Sound of Philadelphia)," the theme to *Soul Train.*

The **8** **Wilma Theater** is named after a Virginia Woolf character. Its unique signage looks especially striking at dusk.

Robinson Luggage, one of the city's last family-owned specialty stores when it closed in 2013, used to occupy the building at S. Broad and Walnut Streets. In a *Philadelphia Inquirer* piece reflecting on the closure, writer Karen Heller, who patronized the store for more than 25 years, described the "old world smell of the place, redolent of leather" and outstanding customer service. After making her last purchase during the going-out-of-business sale, two salespeople hugged her. "Amazon," Heller wrote, "has never once given me anything close to a hug."

The PNB Building (1 S. Broad St.) formerly housed Philadelphia National Bank. The Art Deco high-rise's 17-ton bell rings hourly Monday–Saturday to honor department store magnate John Wanamaker.

City Hall is across the street. There's an old joke that "Broad Street is a straight street—until it gets to City Hall and gets crooked." The South Broad Street II walk starts there.

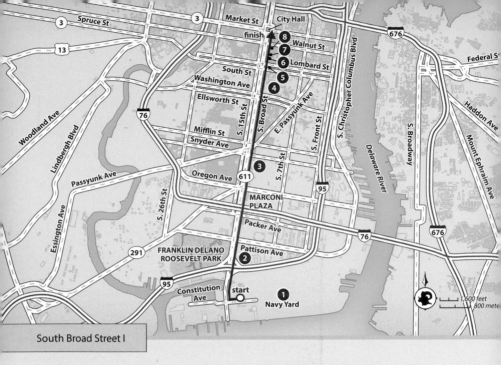

Points of Interest

1 **Philadelphia Navy Yard** 4747 S. Broad St., 215-843-9273, navyyard.org

2 **South Philadelphia Sports Complex** 3300 S. Seventh St.

3 **South Philadelphia High School** 2101 S. Broad St.

4 **Philadelphia High School for Creative and Performing Arts (CAPA)** 901 S. Broad St., 215-400-8140, capa.philasd.org

5 *Theatre of Life* 507 S. Broad St.

6 **University of the Arts Lightbox Film Center** 401 S. Broad St., 215-717-6477, lightboxfilmcenter.org

7 **Broad Street Ministry** 315 S. Broad St., 215-735-4847, broadstreetministry.org

8 **Wilma Theater** 265 S. Broad St., 215-893-9456, wilmatheater.org

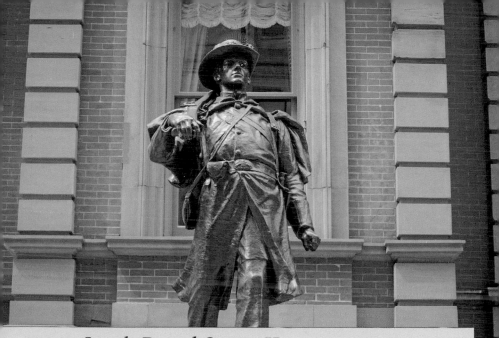

11 South Broad Street II
From the Avenue of the Arts to Franklin Delano Roosevelt Park

Above: The Spirit of '61, in front of The Union League, shows a bronze soldier from the First Regiment Infantry National Guard.

BOUNDARIES: S. Broad St., S. 15th St., Market St., Pattison Ave.
DISTANCE: 3.9 miles
DIFFICULTY: Moderate
PARKING: Driving around here can be tricky, and parking is difficult. Public transportation is the way to get to City Hall.
PUBLIC TRANSIT: The SEPTA subway system is footsteps away, and public buses stop at multiple points around City Hall. Bus 38 stops here and at Independence Hall, the Franklin Institute, and the art museum. Bus 21 travels Walnut St. going west, then returns on Chestnut St. going east. Another option is the PHLASH tourist bus, which operates May–October. Tickets are $2 per ride or $5 for a day pass (free for adults ages 65 and over and for children ages 4 and under).

Broad Street is one of the country's earliest planned roads, developed in 1681 and imagined as "a unifying government and religious center of the new world metropolis." Still, as late as the mid-1800s, this stretch was rural, with businesses and residents concentrated along the Delaware River to the east. Planners built the Academy of Music here in 1857 because it was quiet and remote.

This later became the city's Wall Street, with financial giants including Drexel Company, Girard Trust, and Fidelity Bank building here. Residential development followed, and the mansions of what was once Millionaire's Row still stand, although they've been subdivided into smaller apartments and businesses.

In the 1990s, Mayor Ed Rendell, later governor of Pennsylvania, pushed for the creation of the Avenue of the Arts Inc., a nonprofit organization focused on attracting performing arts groups as well as retail and restaurants. Where there was once a single theatre, now there are four, as well as an expanded University of the Arts, high-end hotels, and restaurants.

Walk Description

Begin at City Hall, where South Broad and Penn Square meet. Critics called the building "the white elephant" when it was completed in 1901 because the marble facade shone so brightly. Take the crosswalk south to the center median; turn slightly right, then cross again. The Ritz-Carlton, Philadelphia (10 Avenue of the Arts) is in the former Girard Bank building.

French-born Stephen Girard, who founded his eponymous bank in 1811, was the richest man in the US when he died in 1831, a billionaire in today's dollars. He put his cash to good use: He kept the country solvent during the War of 1812. He was also a philanthropist: During the yellow fever epidemics of 1793 and 1797, Girard stayed in the city to care for the sick. In his will, he permanently endowed Girard College, a boarding school for "poor, male, white orphans." The school today is co-ed and open to students of all colors.

Continue south. The Land Title Building and Annex (100 S. Broad St.) is one of the country's earliest skyscrapers, the first of its two towers rising 16 stories in 1898. The other, 21 stories tall, was completed a few years later.

Continue to ❶ The Union League of Philadelphia, a members-only club founded in 1862 by supporters of President Abraham Lincoln. It occupies an entire city block.

Outside, the sculpture at right is *Washington Grays Monument,* also known as *Pennsylvania Volunteer,* a tribute to an 1822 volunteer military regiment that served in times of war and peace, similar to today's National Guard. In 1848, the Grays guarded President John Quincy Adams as he lay in state at Independence Hall.

At left is *The Spirit of '61,* a bronze soldier from the First Regiment Infantry National Guard of Philadelphia. It was the first unit called to action in 1861 after the attack on Fort Sumter.

Continue walking south to 200 S. Broad Street. Formerly the Bellevue-Stratford Hotel, the building now houses the Bellevue Hotel, a shopping mall, and offices. Called the "Grande Dame of Broad Street" when it opened in 1904, the Bellevue-Stratford's notable guests included members of the Astor, Morgan, and Vanderbilt families. The 1936 and 1948 Republican National Conventions were held here, as was the 1948 Democratic National Convention. The hotel's fortune changed in 1976 when it was the site of the first known outbreak of Legionnaire's Disease.

Continue on South Broad Street. Next to the hotel is Masayrk Place, named for Tomas Masayrk, the first president of the Czechoslovak Republic. In 1918, Masayrk declared the country's independence in Philadelphia after winning over President Woodrow Wilson during a US visit.

Cross Walnut Street. Look down. Philadelphia Music Alliance's Walk of Fame begins here. Since 1987, more than 100 plaques have been installed to honor local music greats, including Dizzy Gillespie, Billie Holiday, John Coltrane, Marian Anderson, The Roots, and Pearl Bailey. The 2019 inductees included The Hooters and The O'Jays.

Look for the plaque honoring pop/rock duo Hall & Oates, then consider dialing the "Callin' Oates" hotline at 719-26-OATES (719-266-2837). Still active in the summer of 2022, the hotline offers callers the opportunity to hear four of the band's biggest hits. Press 1 for "One on One," 2 for "Rich Girl," 3 for "Maneater," and 4 for "Private Eyes."

Cross Locust Street. The block is also called Patti LaBelle Way. The Philadelphia-born "Godmother of Soul" came to fame in 1970s when her eponymous group released "Lady Marmalade" and became the first African American vocal group on the cover of *Rolling Stone*.

Continue to the ❷ **Academy of Music**. The so-called "Grand Old Lady of Locust Street" is the country's oldest opera house still used for its original purpose. President Franklin Pierce attended its 1855 groundbreaking. Giuseppe Verdi's *Il Trovatore* was the first production. Pyotr Tchaikovsky and Igor Stravinsky performed here in the 19th century, while stars such as Frank Sinatra, Duke Ellington, and Lynn Fontanne did so in the 20th century. Presidents Ulysses S. Grant, Grover Cleveland, and Richard Nixon attended productions. The building is reportedly haunted: women seated in the upper balconies have reported being pinched or having their hair pulled by unseen entities.

The Shubert family built Merriam Theater (250 S. Broad St.) in 1918 to honor a brother killed in a train accident. The University of the Arts, which owns the building, uses it for student activities.

The 21-story Atlantic Building (260 S. Broad St.), constructed in the 1920s for the Atlantic Richfield Oil Refining Company, is now a mixed-use building.

The $180 million ❸ **Kimmel Center for the Performing Arts** is the home of the Philadelphia Orchestra. Built in 2001, it's named for philanthropist Sidney Kimmel, who donated more than $15 million toward its construction.

Next door, the University of the Arts Dorrance Hamilton Hall (320 S. Broad St.) was completed in 1826 for the Pennsylvania School for the Deaf. It's Broad Street's oldest extant building.

Continue south. ❹ **Symphony House/Suzanne Roberts Theatre** is a 32-story mixed-use tower named for the wife of Comcast's founder. Built in 2007, it replaced a gas station and parking lot. Still, architecture critic Inga Saffron called it "the ugliest new condo building in Philadelphia," noting its "mixed-use tower flounces onto venerable South Broad Street like a sequined and over-rouged strumpet." The Philadelphia Theatre Company, based here, is well respected.

The city public health buildings at 500 S. Broad Street stand on the former site of the Dunbar Theater. Businessmen E. C. Brown and Andrew Stevens Jr. opened the theater in 1919 as a showplace for African American performers after Brown was denied entry to the Forrest Theatre because of his skin color. The pair owned one of the most successful African American banks north of the Mason-Dixon line.

The Dunbar, under various owners and a different name, thrived until the Great Depression, hosting some of the country's top African American entertainers, including Lena Horne and Duke Ellington. The building was torn down in 1966.

The ❺ **Philadelphia Clef Club of Jazz and Performing Arts** was the social club of Local 274, the African American musicians' union founded in 1935 by musicians barred from joining a whites-only union. (The original club stood two blocks south at 914 S. Broad Street, now a fast-food restaurant.) The Clef Club relocated here in 1995. It offers performances and music education.

The road between South Street and Washington Avenue honors Reverend Charles A. Tindley, who helmed the still-active Tindley Temple United Methodist Church (750–762 S. Broad St.). Born in 1851 to enslaved parents, Tindley learned to read and write while working as a janitor at Bainbridge Street Methodist Episcopal Church, where he would eventually lead the congregation. He was a civil rights leader and is considered the father of gospel music, credited with composing "Stand by Me" and other hymns. The church says he wrote the lyrics to "We Shall Overcome."

❻ **Circle Mission Church** is owned by the International Peace Mission Movement, founded by Father Major Jealous Divine, a charismatic, sectarian religious leader whose movement took shape in the 1930s. He preached modesty and moral living, urging followers to pool resources and embrace racial integration. Critics called the church a cult. These three buildings were purchased in 1939. Before that, the twin Victorian homes at the corner were a hotel.

The Sprouts Farmers Market (1000 S. Broad St.) is in the former Philadelphia, Wilmington and Baltimore Railroad's circa 1852 restored train shed. The neighboring nine-story mixed-use building covers the rest of the land that housed the city's first passenger train station. Civil War soldiers left from here for points south. President Lincoln's funeral train stopped briefly en route to Illinois.

Cross Washington Avenue. Marine Club Condominiums (1100 S. Broad St.) was the Marine Quartermaster's Depot, which made soldiers' uniforms during the World Wars.

The stretch between Washington and Oregon Avenues is the Avenue of the States, featuring two flags from each state. During the 2016 Democratic National Convention, protesters surrounded Mississippi's flag while shouting "Take it down! Take it down!" The flag included the Confederate battle flag's stars and bars. City officials obliged. In 2021, Mississippi adopted a new flag without Confederate symbols. It flies here today.

The ❼ **National Shrine of St. Rita of Cascia and St. Rita's Church** honors the Italian nun known as the Saint of the Impossible and the Peacemaker. Built in 14th-century Renaissance style, the shrine began as a church for Italian immigrants.

The JNA Culinary Institute of Art (1212 S. Broad St.), now closed, was the 650-seat Dante Theatre, which opened in 1937 and offered Italian-language films.

Continue south. The 40-foot-tall painting of opera singer Mario Lanza (1326 S. Broad St.) shows him midtune, wearing a white bow tie and black tails. The artist listened to Lanza's music while painting.

Cross Reed Street. The City Council renamed this block Jimmy Tayoun Way to honor a former member of the City Council and the Pennsylvania House of Representatives who resigned to spend 40 months in prison after pleading guilty to racketeering, mail fraud, tax evasion, and obstruction of justice charges.

Continue on South Broad. HIVE Café (1444 S. Broad St.) has an outdoors community food pantry installed in 2020 to aid families struggling during the COVID-19 pandemic.

Cross Dickinson Street and continue south. *South Philly Musicians Remix* (1532 S. Broad St.) showcases local musicians, including Chubby Checker, Al Martino, Bobby Rydell, and Fabian.

Continue on South Broad Street. The statue in front of the South Philadelphia Health and Literary Center (1700 S. Broad St.) is South Philadelphia native Evelyn Keyser's *Mother and Child/See the Moon,* installed as part of the 1959 city ordinance requiring that 1% of construction funds for new buildings be spent on fine arts. The Association for Public Art says Keyser wanted to convey "the great affection and protection a mother gives an infant."

Need a break? Take a right on Passyunk Avenue, walk one block to South 15th Street, then turn left. **❽ Melrose Diner** has been open around the clock since 1935 (except during the COVID-19 pandemic). It promotes itself with a jingle that includes, "Everybody who knows goes to Melrose."

Continue south to the former Bell Telephone Company building (2000 S. Broad St.), which fittingly now houses Verizon. Bell Telephone was founded in 1877 with Alexander Graham Bell as chief electrician.

Cross Jackson Street. Most of the block has original structures. Renzetti & Magnarelli Clergy (2216 S. Broad St.) "has been serving the vesturing needs of various religious orders and church organizations for over 50 years," its website notes.

Continue south. The Philadelphia High School for Creative and Performing Arts (2600 S. Broad St.) is better known as CAPA. Alums include Boyz II Men, Leslie Odom Jr., and members of The Roots.

Cross Oregon Avenue. Marconi Plaza is a 19-acre park named for Guglielmo Marconi, who created the wireless telegraph and unidirectional radio. The descriptive plaque at the corner describes Marconi as a "deeply religious humanitarian genius, glory of the world in Italy, and glory of Italy in the world . . . His inventions saved millions of lives and will continue to do so as long as this world exists." The city's Italian American community gathered here to celebrate Italy's World Cup win in 2006.

The multiblock stretch that follows has little of note. Passing the highway on-ramps, check out the statue of Walt Whitman, midstride, hat in hand.

Continue south. After crossing Hartranft Street, the wall of greenery that stretches to Pattison Avenue hides the NovaCare Complex and Field House (2 NovaCare Way), the Philadelphia Eagles' practice field and business offices. Lincoln Financial Field, where the team plays home games, is part of the South Broad Street I walk.

Cross Pattison Avenue to reach **❾ Franklin Delano Roosevelt Park.** This 348-acre oasis includes a golf course, tennis courts, a boathouse, and a gazebo. Its baseball field is named for Richie Ashburn, an All-Star Philadelphia Phillies second baseman who played between 1948 and 1959 and later became a Phillies broadcaster. An overhaul scheduled for completion in 2023 will add a welcome center with food vendors and bathrooms.

Also inside the park is the **❿ American Swedish Historical Museum.** Designed to resemble a 17th-century Swedish castle, the museum opened in the 1920s and is a tribute to the Swedish influence in the area, which dates back the 1600s. Swedes pioneered a building technique that later took over the American frontier: the log cabin.

Explore the opposite side of South Broad Street with Walk 10 (page 59), which begins at the Navy Yard.

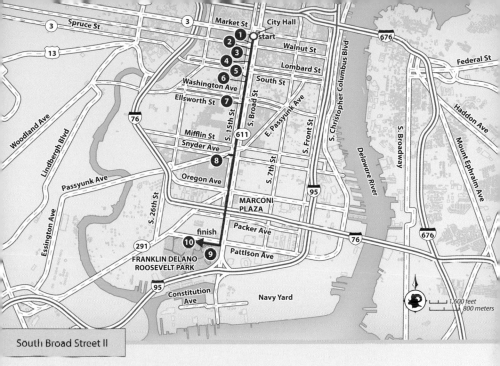

Points of Interest

1. **The Union League of Philadelphia** 140 S. Broad St., 215-563-6500, unionleague.org

2. **Academy of Music** 240 S. Broad St., 215-893-1999, kimmelculturalcampus.org

3. **Kimmel Center for the Performing Arts** 300 S. Broad St., 215-670-2300, kimmelculturalcampus.org

4. **Symphony House/Suzanne Roberts Theatre** 440 S. Broad St., 215-985-1400, philadelphiatheatre-company.org

5. **Philadelphia Clef Club of Jazz and Performing Arts** 738 S. Broad St., 215-893-9912, clefclubofjazz.org

6. **Circle Mission Church** 764–772 S. Broad St., 215-735-3917

7. **National Shrine of St. Rita of Cascia and St. Rita's Church** 1166 S. Broad St., 215-546-8333, saintritashrine.org

8. **Melrose Diner** 1501 Snyder Ave., 215-467-6644, themelrosedinerandbakery.com

9. **Franklin Delano Roosevelt Park** 1500 Pattison Ave., fdrparkphilly.org

10. **American Swedish Historical Museum** 1900 Pattison Ave., 215-389-1776, americanswedish.org

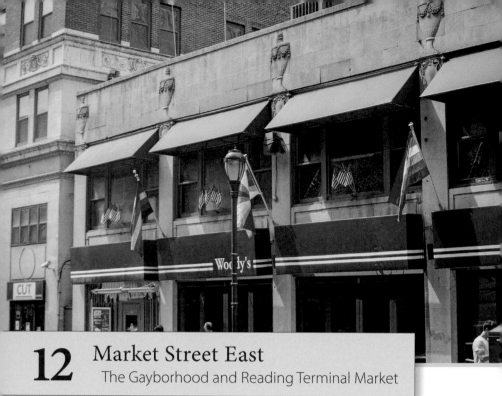

12 Market Street East
The Gayborhood and Reading Terminal Market

Above: Woody's is a well-known Gayborhood nightspot.

BOUNDARIES: Arch St., Pine St., Juniper St., Eighth St.
DISTANCE: 2 miles
DIFFICULTY: Easy
PARKING: While there is some metered street parking, it's hard to get. There are many paid lots. Read signage carefully, as some offer discounts if purchases are made at Reading Terminal Market.
PUBLIC TRANSIT: This tour begins near SEPTA's Jefferson station, and both the Broad Street and Market-Frankford Lines stop here. Buses that stop nearby include the 17, 23, 33, 38, 44, 61, and 78.

Almost every English-speaking town in the 1600s had a shopping thoroughfare called High Street. Philadelphia was no exception. High Street was changed to Market Street in the mid-1800s.

Market Street remains a commercial stretch dotted with historic sites. Many of Benjamin Franklin's activities were centered around Market Street, President George Washington lived on the road, and Thomas Jefferson wrote the Declaration of Independence while renting lodging here.

Walk Description

Begin on the east side of City Hall in front of the statue of John Wanamaker, inscribed with his name and *Citizen*. Founder of the eponymous department store chain, Wanamaker amassed a fortune and generously shared that wealth. He helped build Presbyterian Hospital, cofounded the Sunday Breakfast Rescue Mission to feed the homeless and hungry, and gave to causes, including Irish famine relief and help for victims of the 1913 Ohio River flood. When he died in 1922, public schools were closed and flags lowered to half-mast. About 4,000 residents contributed the $35,000 needed to install this statue.

Cross Juniper Street. The marker on the island at Market and Juniper Streets remembers Philadelphian Anna Jarvis, who founded Mother's Day in 1908. Jarvis said it was Mother's Day, not Mothers' Day, as individuals honored their own maternal figures. Jarvis became angry as the holiday became commercialized. The website explorepahistory.com notes she "objected to greeting cards as 'a poor excuse for the letter you are too lazy to write,' and the sale of flowers and gifts for 'Mother' as turning a day of 'sentiment' into one of 'profit.'" Until her death in 1948, Jarvis fought to reclaim the day, dying penniless.

Cross to the southeast corner of Market Street. Macy's is housed in the ❶ **Wanamaker Building,** formerly Wanamaker's department store. President William Taft attended the December 1911 dedication of the original store, which had five sales floors, each the equivalent of three football fields. The airy marble Grand Court features the Wanamaker Organ, first displayed at the 1904 St. Louis World's Fair. It also holds the eagle, a 2,500-pound bronze statue from the same World's Fair. Generations of shoppers have told friends to "meet me at the eagle." The store's Christmas Light Show has drawn crowds since 1956. Wanamaker's, then and now, is referenced in pop culture. John Travolta's jeep crashes into a window in 1981's *Blow Out*. A character on HBO's *The Sopranos* says he met his wife at the tie counter.

Turn right onto South 13th Street. St. John the Evangelist Catholic Church (21 S. 13th St.), one of the city's busiest parishes, was chartered in 1839. The church once offered a Sunday 2:45 a.m. service to accommodate newspaper employees leaving work around that time.

The ghost sign above Old Nelson Food Co. reads, LADIES AND CHILDREN'S HAIR DRESSING in beautiful script. Civil War veteran Richard Binder opened a hair-dressing parlor here in 1888 when most people had their hair cut at home. He advertised his shop by saying it was close to Wanamaker's.

Cross Chestnut Street, entering Washington Square West—aka Midtown Village, aka the Gayborhood. Long the epicenter of the city's LGBT cultural scene, this formerly run-down, nine-block pocket is a popular dining and entertainment destination. Philadelphia is one of the nation's most gay-friendly cities. In 2003, it actively sought LGBTQ tourists with the tagline "Get your history straight and your nightlife gay." After the U.S. Supreme Court's 2015 decision allowing same-sex marriage, the city's tourism office released the statement "Brotherly or sisterly, love is love."

At left is the DeLong Building, 1232 Chestnut St., which has ornate fire escapes that must be seen to be believed. Completed in the late 1890s, it's named for Frank DeLong, who created an improved hook and eye clothing closure and had his factory here. DeLong is also credited with creating an improved bobby pin.

Stop at Drury Street. At 102 S. 13th Street is a mural of urban planner and visionary Edmund Bacon, "The Father of Modern Philadelphia." He's also the father of actor Kevin. Look left down the alley. ❷ **McGillin's Olde Ale House,** the city's oldest continuously operating tavern, was opened in 1860 by Irish immigrants Catherine and William McGillin. They raised their 13 children in an upstairs apartment. Ma McGillin, who ran the bar until dying in 1937, still haunts the premises.

Cross Walnut Street. This stretch of South 13th Street is Edie Windsor Way, named for the plaintiff in the U.S. Supreme Court case that found parts of the 1996 Defense of Marriage Act unconstitutional. Windsor sued the U.S. government in 2010 following the death of her wife, Thea Spyer, after the government tried to collect $600,000 in inheritance taxes because their Canadian union was not recognized. The case was a significant step forward in the fight for marriage equality.

❸ **Woody's** is a bustling bar and restaurant that the city's official promotional materials describe this way: "Paris has the Eiffel Tower, and London Big Ben, and the Gayborhood has Woody's, a neighborhood landmark since 1980."

Continue south. On Chancellor Street, at left, is a bright wall painting of cockatoo wings that invites selfies. Farther down the street is ❹ **Franky Bradley's,** (1320 Chancellor St.), a bar/restaurant opened in 1933 by retired boxer Franky Bloch, who called himself Bradley professionally. The gayborhoodguru.wordpress.com writes, "It was common at that time for Jewish prizefighters to use Irish names."

Pause at South 13th and Locust Streets. This stretch is named for Barbara Gittings, the mother of the LGBT civil rights movement. With Frank Kameny, the movement's father, she organized early gay rights marches and challenged the American Psychiatric Association's position that homosexuality was a mental illness. The Association changed the classification in 1973, prompting Kameny to quip it was the day "we were cured en masse by psychiatrists." Gittings edited the nation's first lesbian publication and advocated for more gay and lesbian literature in libraries.

Philadelphia Muses celebrates creative expression. Nest (1301 Locust St.) is testament to the area's changes: 10 years ago, this property was a strip club. Before that, it was a XXX movie center. Today, it's a children's activity center.

The Historical Society of Pennsylvania is at 1300 Locust Street. Dedicated in 1910, the building is completely fireproof, as is fitting of a structure holding more than 300 years of historic documents.

Continue south. A historic marker at 233 S. 13th Street recognizes the *Philadelphia Gay News'* first offices. PGN founder Mark Segal is a longtime LGBTQ rights activist, who in 1969 took part in New York's Stonewall Inn uprising, then interrupted Walter Cronkite's nightly newscast by standing in front of the camera with a sign reading, "Gays Protest CBS News Prejudice." He was removed from the set, but he'd piqued Cronkite's interest. As *Smithsonian* reports, "Less than six months later, CBS Evening News featured a segment on gay rights. . . . 'Part of the new morality of the '60s and '70s is a new attitude toward homosexuality,' Cronkite told viewers."

John C. Anderson Apartments (251 S. 13th St.) is Pennsylvania's first LGBTQ-friendly apartment building, named for a city councilperson who died of AIDS in 1983. PGN's Segal conceived of the project for "the first out generation."

Continue south, crossing Spruce Street. Church of St. Luke & the Epiphany (330 S. 13th St.) is an Episcopal parish proud of its diverse congregation. Its website notes, "The Church belongs to God in Christ and therefore anyone whom God brings here, belongs here."

At Pine Street, turn left. **5** **Giovanni's Room,** named for a 1956 James Baldwin book, is the country's oldest gay and lesbian bookstore.

At South 12th Street, turn left. At Spruce Street, turn left.

At South Camac Street, also called Avenue of the Artists, turn right. **6** **The Plastic Club** was founded in 1897 by women artists who challenged the idea that only men could be professional artists. Men joined in the 1990s and today make up about half the membership. The club continues to advance the visual arts, offering exhibitions and lectures.

Neighboring **7** **Tavern on Camac** may be the city's oldest continuously operating gay bar, opening in the 1920s as Maxine's, a gay-friendly speakeasy. One longtime bartender/patron was Mary the Hat. As *The Philadelphia Gayborhood Guru* (thegayborhoodguru.wordpress.com) writes, Mary, who died in 1984, lived in an apartment across the alley. On rainy nights, when she'd call a cab, the driver would park in front of the bar and open the passenger's side back door. Mary would slide in. The driver would then open the driver's side back door and help Mary to her apartment.

The house at 239 S. Camac Street was the Charlotte Cushman Club, founded in 1907 to provide safe and reasonably priced accommodations for visiting actresses. A local theater patron created the club after overhearing two young actresses talk about the unwanted male attention they received in city hotels.

⑧ The Philadelphia Sketch Club, founded in 1860 by six Pennsylvania Academy of Fine Arts students, one time offered classes by artist Thomas Eakins. It remains a gathering place for artists and their supporters.

At Locust Street, turn right. The Princeton Club formerly inhabited 1221 and 1223 Locust Street, two private homes built in the1890s.

At South 12th Street, turn left. This is also Gloria Casarez Way, named for the city's first director of LGBT affairs who was integral to the city's adoption of a groundbreaking LGBT Equality Bill.

The building at 219 S. 12th Street was once part of the SS White Company, makers of high-quality dental products. White, a dentist, began making false teeth from feldspar, a common rock-forming mineral, in the 1840s. A 1918 White toothpaste advertisement in *The Saturday Evening Post* boasted that "American Teeth Impress Our British Allies" and includes an article from a UK newspaper with the headline "U.S. Teeth."

Continue on South 12th Street to Walnut Street. At right is the Beasley Building (1125 Walnut St.), a 19th-century Episcopal Church that in the 1970s became Philadelphia's version of New York's Studio 54. The disco lovers were evicted in 1986 when the property was sold to personal injury lawyers. Temple University Law School is named for founding partner Jim Beasley, whose biography is *Courtroom Cowboy*.

Reading Terminal Market offers fresh meat, fish, and produce and prepared delights from around the world.

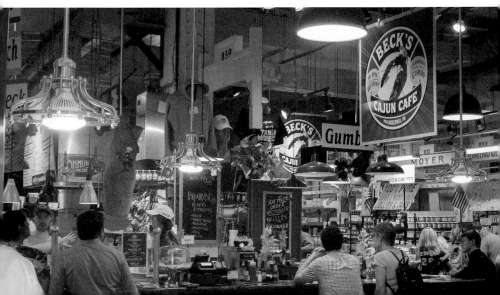

9 **Finn McCools Ale House** is named for a giant who threw rocks between the Irish and Scottish coasts so he could walk across to fight with a Scottish rival. The result: Giant's Causeway, a World Heritage site.

Turn right on Sansom Street. Walk to *The Promise of Biotechnology* (1108 Sansom St.) and turn around. Artist Amy Sherald, perhaps best known for her portrait of Michelle Obama, painted *Untitled* (1108 Sansom St.) in 2019. The girl depicted in the six-story-tall work was part of Mural Arts Philadelphia's Youth Education Program.

Return to Finn McCools and turn right, walking north and passing Drexel University's Kline Institute of Trial Advocacy (1200 Chestnut St.). The Beneficial Savings Fund Society, which opened in 1918, catered to immigrants. A century later, it was outfitted with five authentic courtrooms to stage mock trials.

Continue to Market Street. **10** **Loews Philadelphia Hotel** was built in 1933 for the Philadelphia Savings Fund Society. The glowing PSFS letters atop the building were an oddity at the time. The bank kept the letters lit during the Great Depression to reassure customers their bank was secure. (Some said the letters actually meant "Philadelphia Slowly Facing Starvation.") Loews, which opened in 2000, maintains the sign.

This was also the site of America's first circus, Ricketts Circus. In 1793, British equestrian John Bill Ricketts built a horse ring, where he performed riding tricks for paying customers. As his show's popularity grew, Ricketts added other performers, including tightrope walkers, jugglers, and clowns. President George Washington was a fan, allowing Ricketts to display his own white steed, Jack, in the building. Ricketts marked Washington's 1797 retirement with a farewell show, then months later welcomed President John Adams to another performance. In 1799, a fire destroyed the theater. Brokenhearted, Ricketts left town.

Continue north. The Reading Terminal Building (1115–1141 Market St.) was built in the 1880s to rival Pennsylvania Railroad's fortresslike station nearby. The first train departed from here in 1893; the last, in 1984.

Pass Filbert Street and come to **11** **Reading Terminal Market.** When the railroad completed its terminal, it provided space on the train shed's ground floor for 800 vendors. The market thrived until the early 1970s. A few years later, the building was falling apart and only 23 merchants remained.

The Pennsylvania Convention Center purchased the space in the 1990s. Today it's a local favorite and a must-visit tourist attraction, with 80 independently owned businesses. *Philbert,* the pig statue inside, invites visitors to rub his snout for good luck. (Promotional materials call him "the Market's favorite pork product not topped with broccoli rabe and provolone.") Coins dropped into Philbert's base support a local food charity. Philbert is in a long-term, long-distance relationship with *Rachel*, a similar sculpture at Seattle's Pike Place Market.

At Arch Street, turn right. The ⑫ **Pennsylvania Convention Center** occupies four city blocks. Opened in 1993, it underwent a $700 million expansion that was completed in 2011. It hosts about 250 events annually, including the Philadelphia Flower Show, the world's oldest and largest of its kind.

The Pitcairn Building (1027 Arch St.) was erected in 1901 for the Pittsburgh Plate Glass Company. Company founder John Pitcairn Jr. was successful in business, less successful in love. He pursued his future wife for two years until she married him. She died young, leaving four children. Pitcairn didn't remarry, saying, "I would no sooner remarry than if Gertrude were standing in the other room."

At South 11th Street, turn right. ⑬ **Tom's Dim Sum** is known for soup dumplings, even if one food writer described the decor as "the offspring between a well-off suburban Italian bistro and a Shanghai Chipotle franchise. Plus neon."

At Market Street, turn left. The city's Fashion District, unveiled in 2019, stretches from N. 11th to N. 7th Streets. It averaged 700,000 visitors per month in its first year. Stores can be reached via the street or from its mall, which has entrances at 9th and 10th Streets.

Continue east. The Robert N. C. Nix Federal Building (900 Market St.), named for the first African American to represent Pennsylvania in Congress, was built in the 1930s as a Public Works Administration project, as the building's bas-reliefs attest.

The now-closed Strawbridge & Clothier (801 Market St.) started as a dry-goods store founded in 1868 by Quakers Justus Strawbridge and Isaac Clothier with the motto, "Small profits, one price, for cash only." It grew to fill this 13-story Beaux Arts structure built in 1928.

The Lit Brothers department store occupied 701–739 Market Street, an assemblage of 11 buildings. Samuel and Jacob Lit marketed their store as "A Great Store in a Great City" that was less expensive than Strawbridge & Clothier. The store closed in 1977, but the Lit Brothers name still encircles the property, promising "Hats Trimmed Free of Charge."

Continue east. This walk's last stop is ⑭ **Declaration House**, a reconstruction of the home where Thomas Jefferson wrote the Declaration of Independence. Jefferson rented two furnished second-floor rooms, re-created here, including a replica of the small bed into which he squeezed his 6-foot-2 frame. Jefferson complained the nearby stables attracted horseflies that bothered him as he wrote.

Other tours begin at Washington Square, a few blocks south, and Independence Visitor Center, a few blocks east.

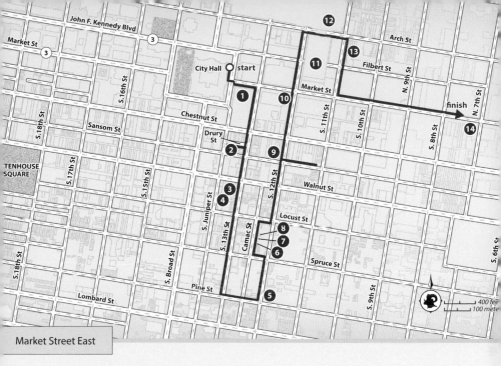

Points of Interest

1. **Wanamaker Building (now Macy's)** 1300 Market St., 215-241-9000, macys.com
2. **McGillin's Olde Ale House** 1310 Drury St., 215-735-5562, mcgillins.com
3. **Woody's** 202 S. 13th St., 215-545-1893, woodysbar.com
4. **Franky Bradley's** 1320 Chancellor St., 215-735-0735, frankybradleys.com
5. **Giovanni's Room** 345 S. 12th St., 215-923-2960, queerbooks.com
6. **The Plastic Club** 247 S. Camac St., 215-545-9324, plasticclub.org
7. **Tavern on Camac** 243 S. Camac St., 215-545-0900, tavernoncamac.com
8. **The Philadelphia Sketch Club** 235 S. Camac St., 215-545-9298, sketchclub.org
9. **Finn McCools Ale House** 118 S. 12th St., 215-923-3090, finnmccoolsphilly.com
10. **Loews Philadelphia Hotel** 1200 Market St., 215-627-1200, loewshotels.com
11. **Reading Terminal Market** 51 N. 12th St., 215-922-2317, readingterminalmarket.org
12. **Pennsylvania Convention Center** 1101 Arch St., 215-418-4700, paconvention.com
13. **Tom's Dim Sum** 59 N. 11th St., 215-923-8880, tomsdimsum.com
14. **Declaration House** 599 S. Seventh St., 215-965-2305, nps.gov/inde

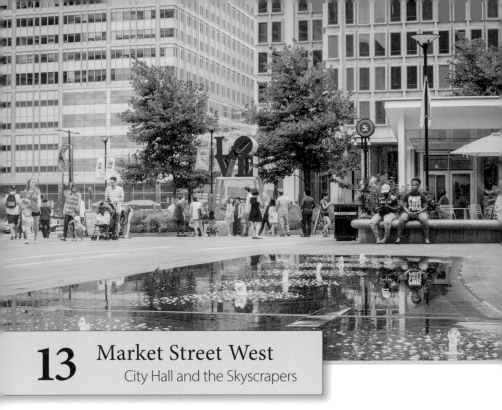

13 Market Street West
City Hall and the Skyscrapers

Above: Dilworth Plaza, on the west side of City Hall, features programmed water jets that cool residents in summer.

BOUNDARIES: S. 13th St., N. 18th St., John F. Kennedy Blvd., Chestnut St.
DISTANCE: 1 mile
DIFFICULTY: Easy
PARKING: Metered street parking is tough. Pay lots are available.
PUBLIC TRANSIT: The best way to reach City Hall is on foot or by using public transportation. Nearby subway stops include City Hall and Suburban Station. Buses include the 16 and the 31.

When Philadelphia City Hall opened in 1901 after 30 years of construction, it became the city's tallest building, with its bell tower topped with a 37-foot-tall likeness of William Penn by Alexander Milne Calder.

For decades, no building was made higher than the top of Penn's hat. Some thought to do so would violate a gentleman's agreement between the city and local builders. When One and Two Liberty Place broke that agreement in 1987, the curse of Billy Penn began. This tour tells that story.

Walk Description

Start at **❶ City Hall.** The compass at the center courtyard, featuring zodiac signs and compass points in gold leaf, marks the exact city center established by William Penn in the 1600s. The compass was a 1984 gift from legendary city planner Edmund Bacon, who financed the project by selling a 15th-century illuminated manuscript made by monks.

This ornate building has more than 250 architectural reliefs and sculptures, which is odd in a city founded by simplicity-loving Quakers. It's topped by a 37-foot-tall statue of Penn. His left hand points to Penn Treaty Park, where he signed a peace agreement with the native Lenni Lenape. His right hand holds a rolled-up copy of the Charter of Pennsylvania. From certain angles, that scroll makes it appear Penn is standing at a urinal.

City Hall appears in movies, including *Trading Places, Twelve Monkeys,* and *Philadelphia.*

Exit the courtyard via the west exit, guided by the compass. Dilworth Park, named for a former mayor, was wasted space until a 2014 renovation. Additions included programmable fountains that shoot straight from the ground, a café, a performance and market space, and new glass-encased entrances to the city's subway system. In the winter, the fountains become an ice rink.

Turn left. Walk to the park's southwest corner. Across the street is Robert Engman's *Triune,* installed in 1975. The name means "three in one." Engman said the three bronze curves represent people, government, and business.

Across the street to the right is **❷ The Clothespin,** a 45-foot-tall steel structure by Claes Oldenburg, who took inspiration from Gustav Klimt's *The Kiss.*

Use the crosswalk at right to walk west on Market Street. Pass 1515 Market, then turn around to see *Milord la Chamarre* or *My Lord of the Fancy Vest* by French painter and sculptor Jean Dubuffet, on the second floor. Dubuffet is credited with founding the art brut movement.

Continue on Market Street. **❸ One and Two Liberty Place** were, in 1987, the first buildings taller than William Penn's hat. When the towers were first proposed, a newspaper poll revealed citizens opposed breaking the height barrier by a vote of 3,809 to 1,822. Bacon told *The New York Times* the development would decimate "the scale of Center City." Those opponents sang a different tune when the buildings were completed. The *Philadelphia Inquirer,* which had denounced the project, published a 1990 piece headlined "Taking It All Back, Liberty Place Turned Out to Be a Swell Idea."

It wasn't all swell. Building higher than Penn's hat triggered the "Curse of Billy Penn." Between 1987 and 2007, none of the city's major sports teams won a championship. The curse was broken in June 2007 when, as construction of what would be the city's tallest building (Comcast Center, see below) was ending, a small statue of Penn was affixed to a top beam. Penn was back on top and, thus appeased, allowed the Phillies to win the 2008 World Series.

The city's teams soon sank back into oblivion. In November 2017, when construction began on the Comcast Technology Center, what is now the city's tallest structure, builders "rushed the final steel beams into place over two weeks . . . then affixed a tiny Billy Penn statue (and a Christmas tree) to the highest beam, putting Billy Penn in his rightful place overlooking the city from its highest vantage point," the *Philadelphia Inquirer* reported. "They did not want to take the chance and wait for the jinx," a Comcast executive told the newspaper.

A few months later, the Eagles won the Super Bowl.

Continue on Market Street. The BNY Mellon Center (1735 Market St.), which appears as a backdrop in 1993's *Philadelphia,* is part of the Penn Center complex, a collection of 11 mid- and high-rise buildings stretching from 15th to 19th Streets and Market Street to John F. Kennedy Boulevard. The mixed-use development was considered radical when Bacon proposed it in the 1950s. He later described introducing the development at a Chamber of Commerce meeting, saying the mayor "was so scared he refused to sit at the speaker's table."

At 18th Street, turn right. At John F. Kennedy Boulevard, turn right. At the corner is the Arch Street Presbyterian Church (1724 Arch St.), built in 1855. The neoclassical Greek Revival–style building stands in contrast to ❹ **Comcast Center,** at 58 stories the city's second-tallest building. The city's tallest building, the 60-story Comcast Technology Center, is right next door. Architecture critic Inga Saffron wrote that the former resembles a giant flash drive. On foggy nights, the latter and "its signature switchblade mast looks like something out of Batman's Gotham, mysterious and brooding," she said. Others say the extended mast looks like a middle finger.

At North 17th Street, with the Art Deco wonder that is Suburban Street Station ahead, turn right and cross Market Street. The United Plaza building houses Duane Morris LLP, one of the world's largest law firms, founded in 1904. In front of the building is Roy Lichtenstein's four-part sculpture ❺ *Brushstroke Group.* In 2005, *Philadelphia Inquirer* art critic Edward J. Sozanski compared this work to *The Clothespin,* saying *Brushstroke Group* "is equally witty, more complex visually and, because of its intense colors, far more animated."

Continue on South 17th Street. At Ranstead Street, turn right and enter ❻ **John F. Collins Park**. The gate's details are a tribute to the nearby marshlands of New Jersey and Delaware and include turtles, fish, and birds. The interior fountain is a tribute to Native American totems. Exit via

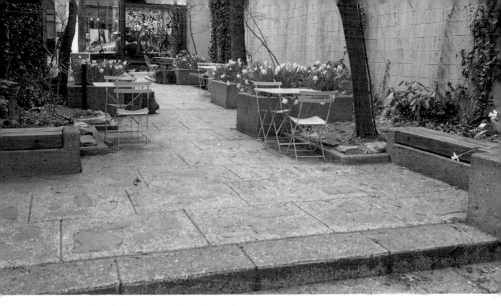

John F. Collins Park is a hidden gem in busy Center City.

the Chestnut Street gate, which is a tribute to the Wissahickon and Delaware Valleys, featuring an owl, flowers, insects, and birds. If the Ranstead Street gate is locked, circle the block to the Chestnut Street exit to pick up the walk again.

The eight-story Art Deco building across the street once housed upscale retailer Bonwit Teller, which closed in 1990 but achieved immortality thanks to Philadelphia's favorite fictional boxer. In 1979's *Rocky II*, Rocky illegally parks next to the store, then runs inside to buy a black satin jacket with a tiger on the back, a fur coat for Adrian, and a watch for Paulie.

Turn left, walking east on Chestnut Street. The Art Deco structure at 1622 Chestnut St., built in 1934, originally housed WCAU, one of the city's first AM radio stations.

Five Below (1529 Chestnut St.) was the Arcadia Theatre, which opened in April 1915 with ticket prices ranging from 15 to 25 cents. The Arcadia closed in 1978 and a fast food restaurant took over the space. Cinematreasures.org said "it was the most interesting fast food place in town. It retained the slope of the theatre, with a ramp to the former stage where the food was sold. The seating was in tiers in the former audience area."

Another movie theater marquee is at 1519 Chestnut Street. This one is . . . a Foot Locker. This was the 500-seat Trans-Lux Theater, which opened in 1934. In 1955, the theater hosted the world premiere of *To Catch a Thief,* an event attended by stars Cary Grant and former local Grace Kelly. Retail moved into the space in the 2000s.

Continue east. The former First Pennsylvania Bank (1426 Chestnut St.) now has a Del Frisco's Double Eagle Steakhouse on its lower floors. Its past is hinted at by the 40-foot black iron front gate and the words "Pennsylvania Building" and "Insurances on lives and granting annuities" carved above the door. Safe-deposit boxes line the restaurant's private dining room. The original bank clock remains above the bar, stopped at 5 o'clock.

The former Jacob Reed's Sons Building (1424 Chestnut St.), finished in 1903, looks like a Northern Italian palazzo, complete with Byzantine mosaics. This building was meant to convey the clothing company's old-fashioned values and attention to detail.

The top of the American Baptist Publication Society (1420–22 Chestnut St.), built in 1896, resembles a French château.

7 **Prince Theater** replaced the Karlton Theatre, which opened on this spot in 1921 with Italian marble floors and fountains. It hosted the world premiere of the movie *Adam's Rib* in 1949 and the world premiere of *Rocky II* in 1979.

Continue toward Broad Street. The marker at 1400 Chestnut Street recognizes politician Anne Brancato Wood, the first female Democrat elected to the Pennsylvania House of Representatives and the first woman to become speaker pro tem. She advocated for women and the poor, taking up causes like child labor protection and minimum wage laws. One of her bills was 1936's Hasty Marriage Act, which required couples to wait three days after applying for a marriage license before marrying. She said that would give women being forced into marriage time to escape.

Continue to The Widener Building (1327–39 Chestnut St.). Philadelphia architect Horace Trumbauer built this in a classical European style with an elaborate arcade. Trumbauer had a long relationship with the wealthy Widener family, who made their fortune from U.S. Steel and the American Tobacco Company. He also designed Harvard University's Widener Library, built to honor a relative who died on the *Titanic*.

A historical marker notes the first American photo, a daguerreotype of Central High School that took 10 minutes to expose, was taken here in 1839. The camera was made from a cigar box and a lens.

This walk ends here. Head to City Hall to begin another tour.

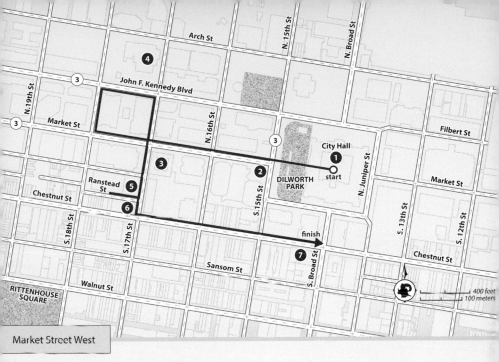

Points of Interest

1 **City Hall** 1401 John F. Kennedy Blvd., 215-686-1776, phila.gov

2 *The Clothespin* 1500 Market St. For more information, contact the Association for Public Art, 215-546-7550, associationforpublicart.org.

3 **One and Two Liberty Place** 1650 Market St., 215-851-9000, onelibertyplace.com

4 **Comcast Center** 1701 John F. Kennedy Blvd., 215-496-1810, comcastcentercampus.com

5 *Brushstroke Group* 30 S. 17th St. For more information, contact the Association for Public Art, 215-546-7550, associationforpublicart.org.

6 **John F. Collins Park** 1707 Chestnut St., 215-440-5500, ccdparks.org/john-f-collins-park

7 **Prince Theater** 1412 Chestnut St., 215-422-4580, princetheater.org

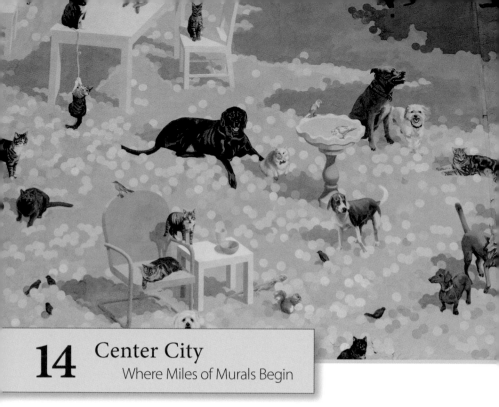

14 Center City
Where Miles of Murals Begin

BOUNDARIES: Market St., South St., S. Seventh St., Broad St.
DISTANCE: About 2.5 miles
DIFFICULTY: Easy
PARKING: This tour begins in the 700 block of Chestnut St. There is a private parking facility on this block, as well as metered parking on the street.
PUBLIC TRANSIT: Multiple buses stop near the 700 block, including the 9 and the 21. If traveling by subway, take the Market-Frankford Line to the Eighth Street Station.

Philadelphia is the Mural Capital of the World, with more than 4,000 city walls painted with larger-than-life works creating a massive outdoor art gallery. The city-affiliated agency behind these works, Mural Arts Philadelphia, believes art can ignite positive change. The program launched in 1984 as the Anti-Graffiti Network, hiring and encouraging local graffiti artists to create something positive with their skills. It was an immediate success, and executive director Jane Golden realized her group wasn't anti anything; it was pro art. Almost 40 years later, Mural Arts Phila-delphia is the nation's largest public art program, partnering with diverse groups for projects throughout the city. The program offers multiple tours, guided and self-guided, on foot, by bike, or via trolley or Segway. This Center City walk is a good introduction to both that program and the city. It includes the so-called "Mural Mile," although this walk's distance is closer to 2.5 miles.

Walk Description

Begin at ❶ *Legacy,* a 4,000-square-foot photo-realistic work honoring Abraham Lincoln that's composed of more than 1 million 0.75-inch glass tiles from Italy and France.

Enter the neighboring parking lot to see more. At left is a map of Africa and a slave ship with iron shackles. Near the center, a girl wears a necklace with three coins: one featuring Lincoln, another Frederick Douglass, and an 1838 British abolitionist coin showing a freed slave and the words, "Am I not a woman and a sister." In the girl's palm, an older version of herself rises through flames, signifying the strength she and her ancestors have shown. The text at lower right comes from the final debate between Lincoln and Stephen Douglas.

Walk west on Chestnut Street. At South Eighth Street, turn right. At Ranstead Street, *A People's Progression towards Equality* also honors Lincoln. The lower portion contains images related to slavery and segregation. At top is an excerpt from the Gettysburg Address: "With malice toward none, with charity for all."

Continue on South Eighth Street. Cross Market Street, then turn left. This is the start of the Fashion District, a concentration of more than 70 stores, dining options, entertainment venues, and art installations unveiled in 2019. It averaged 700,000 visitors per month in its first year. Stores can be reached via the street or from its mall, which also has entrances at Market and 9th Streets and Market and 10th Streets.

Continue on Market Street, crossing 11th Street. This section of the Pennsylvania Convention Center was the Philadelphia and Reading Railroad's passenger terminal, built in 1893. Continue, crossing 12th Street. Note the Loews Hotel on the opposite corner. This was the Philadelphia Savings Fund Society, and the letters PSFS atop the building are still lit nightly.

At 13th Street, ❷ *Tree of Knowledge* was sponsored by the Eisenhower Fellowship, an inter-national exchange program. Ladders help people reach items among the tree branches relat-ing to different fields, such as musical instruments and carpentry tools. A quote from President Dwight D. Eisenhower reads, "Only justice, fairness, consideration and cooperation can finally lead men to the dawn of eternal peace."

At South 13th Street, turn left, crossing Market Street. Before reaching St. John the Evangelist Church, look left. ❸ *Finding Home* aims to erase the stigma of homelessness. Walk down the alley next to the church to fully appreciate the work.

The artists asked homeless individuals to write their stories and struggles on strips of fabric, which were woven to create the mural's canvas. Differently colored hands coming together in prayer symbolize a united community. Mixed in are black-and-white snapshots of happy home lives that many lack.

Continue on South 13th Street. Cross Clover Street. Signage on the second floor of the Old Nelson II Food Company (35 S. 13th St.) reveals this building once housed the Binder Company, hairdressers and makers of wigs, toupees, soaps, and . . . cigars?

At Chestnut Street, turn left. At South 12th Street, turn right, walking around Drexel University's Kline Institute of Trial Advocacy (1200 Chestnut St.), the former Beneficial Savings Fund Society, which opened in 1918 and catered to immigrants. A century later, it was outfitted with five authentic courtrooms to stage mock trials.

Continue on South 12th Street. *Building the City* (S. 12th and Moravian Sts.) features public artworks, including the William Penn statue. At Locust Street, turn left. This stretch is also called Barbara Gittings Way, recognizing the LGBTQ civil rights pioneer. The cross street is Edie Windsor Way, honoring the lead plaintiff in the 2013 Supreme Court decision U.S. v. Windsor, which led to the legalization of same-sex marriage.

At South Sartain Street, ❹ *Garden of Delight* includes trees leaning toward each other as if to embrace. The artist says this work is to be enjoyed, not overanalyzed.

In front of the mural, turn right to walk west on Locust Street. ❺ *Philadelphia Muses* reimagines the nine Muses of Greek mythology as contemporary concepts such as craft and movement. Each Muse is modeled after a local artist. The woman at center worked for the local opera company, while the man lying across the bottom was a Pennsylvania Ballet dancer.

The New Century Guild (1301 Locust St.) was founded in 1882 to highlight women's contributions to society. Pass the building and turn around to see its mural. *Women of Progress* shows Guild founder Eliza Turner atop the staircase. Also featured are Anne Preston, one of the country's first female doctors, and First Lady Eleanor Roosevelt.

Continue west. The historic Dr. Joseph Leidy House (1319 Locust St.) is the headquarters of the National Union of Hospital and Health Care Employees. Among Leidy's accomplishments: Being a CSI pioneer. In 1845, he used a microscope to prove that blood on a murder suspect's shirt wasn't from chickens, as the man claimed, because it lacked an element known to stay in chicken blood after it was spilled. The suspect then confessed.

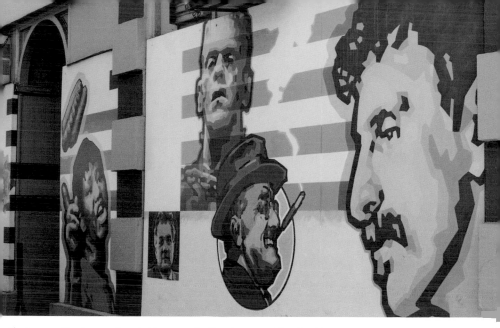

The Famous Franks *mural marks the unmarked bar known as Dirty Frank's.*

At Juniper Street, turn left. ❻ *Pride and Progress*, on the William Way LGBT community center, celebrates the gay rights movement's Philadelphia roots with images of a 1960s-era protest march and a modern gay pride event. Barbara Gittings is at left, wearing a rainbow shirt.

Continue to Spruce Street. At left, ❼ *Taste of Summer* features diners enjoying an outdoor meal. The bald man in the white coat, at far right, is chef Marc Vetri. A girl is based on the daughter of a parking attendant who left his family overseas to work in the US.

Continue on Juniper Street. At Cypress Street, turn left. ❽ **Writer's Block Rehab** is a bar, not a recovery facility. Its west wall shows Alain Locke, the Philadelphia born man called the "father of the Harlem Renaissance." Continue on Cypress to see the opposite wall featuring rapper Lil Nas X, known for 2019's hit "Old Town Road." The images are from the video for 2021's "Montero (Call Me By Your Name)."

Continue on Cypress Street. At South 13th Street, turn right. Ahead is ❾ *Famous Franks*, which marks Dirty Frank's, a local institution. The mural includes St. Francis of Assisi, Aretha Franklin, Frankenstein's monster, Pope Francis, and Phillies legend Tug McGraw, whose actual first name was Frank.

Across the street, David Guinn's *Spring* features towering Bradford pears and dogwoods meant to connect to the real trees bordering the wall.

At Pine Street, turn right. At South Broad Street, turn left. *Theatre of Life,* at Broad and Lombard Streets, is one of the first murals to move beyond two dimensions, incorporating marbles and 3-D masks. Artist Meg Saligman said the mural explores identity and the roles people play. Note the dreamer at left, cutting the strings that control her.

At Lombard Street, turn left. *Gimme Shelter* (1236 Lombard St.), on Morris Animal Refuge, shows pets waiting for forever families. Morris financed the work by selling raffle tickets. Winners' pets are featured in the mural. Look for Butch, a gray tabby whose mom worked at the shelter.

Continue on Lombard Street. Turn right at South 12th Street. At South Street, turn left. ❿ **Philadelphia's Magic Gardens** showcase Isaiah Zagar's distinct works featuring broken tiles, painted figures, and trash turned treasures, including bike tires. Mirror strips send messages or outline drawings. Paying visitors can explore the tunnels and grottoes of the ever-expanding but permanent exhibit.

Continue, turning right on Alder Street for more mosaics. At Bainbridge Street, turn left. ⓫ *Winter: Crystal Snowscape,* at South 10th and Bainbridge Streets, is another in Guinn's Seasons series. The artist is the skier moving toward the light and a bright future.

Continue on Bainbridge Street. The brick building at 915 Bainbridge was the Institute for Colored Youth in 1837.

At South Ninth Street, turn left. At South Street, turn right. Pass 812 South Street, where civil rights leader Octavius Catto, a former Institute for Colored Youth student, lived until his murder in 1871.

Continue east. The electrical box at Greene Street Consignment (700 South St.) is painted with a quote from the late John Lewis, a civil rights pioneer and longtime politician: "Get into good trouble."

Continue to *Mapping Courage: Honoring W. E. B. Du Bois and Engine #11* (South and S. Sixth Sts.), a tribute to Du Bois, the first African American to earn a Harvard University PhD. He's seen in a top hat and tails, which is what he wore while doing his door-to door research here in the late 1800s.

Across from the mural is an electrical box reading, "Bad ass things happen in Philly," a reference to President Donald Trump's statement before the 2020 election that "Bad things happen in Philadelphia." Trump was implying city leaders would cheat to deny him a second term. Coincidentally, Pennsylvania's 20 electoral college votes pushed President Joe Biden to victory.

This walk ends here, as does the African American tour (page 14). Consider following that walk in reverse.

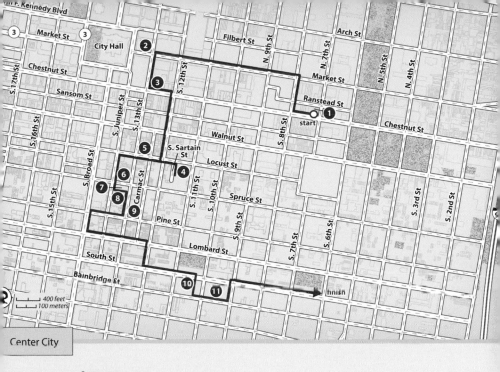

Points of Interest

Unless otherwise noted, call 215-685-0750 or visit muralarts.org for more information.

① *Legacy* 707 Chestnut St.

② *Tree of Knowledge* 1301 Market St.

③ *Finding Home* 21 S. 13th St., wrapped around a building managed by Project H.O.M.E. For information about the nonprofit, call 215-232-7272 or visit projecthome.org.

④ *Garden of Delight* 203 S. Sartain St.

⑤ *Philadelphia Muses* 1235 Locust St.

⑥ *Pride and Progress* 1315 Spruce St.

⑦ *Taste of Summer* 1312 Spruce St

⑧ **Writer's Block Rehab** 1342 Cypress St., 215-603-6960

⑨ *Famous Franks* 347 S. 13th St

⑩ **Philadelphia's Magic Gardens** 1020 South St., 215-733-0390, phillymagicgardens.org

⑪ *Winter: Crystal Snowscape* S. 10th and Bainbridge Sts.

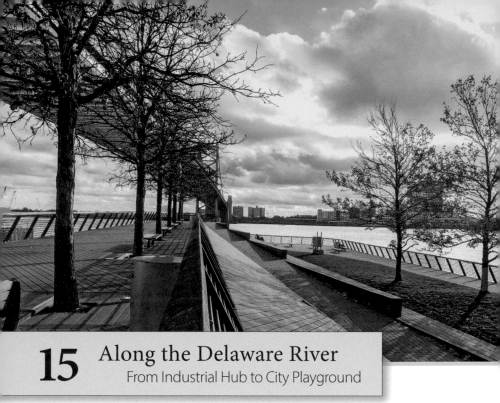

15 Along the Delaware River
From Industrial Hub to City Playground

BOUNDARIES: Delaware River, N. Seventh St., Monroe St., Callowhill St.
DISTANCE: 2 miles
DIFFICULTY: Easy
PARKING: Public lots and street parking are available.
PUBLIC TRANSIT: Multiple SEPTA buses stop nearby, including the 79 and the 25.

Philadelphia is the city it is today because of the Delaware River. When William Penn arrived on its banks, he saw opportunities for commerce and recreation. The first port was built in 1681. By the 1700s, Philadelphia was the second-busiest port in the world, after London.

The waterfront's fortunes began to wane in the 1800s as commerce moved north to New York and further suffered as the city lost its manufacturing base in the mid-1900s. The construction of I-95 in the 1970s further cut off the river.

The waterfront's upswing began in the 1990s and continues. Race Street and Cherry Street Piers and Spruce Street Harbor Park have quickly become local and tourist favorites. The Delaware River Trail, 6 miles of protected bike lanes and a pedestrian sidewalk stretching from Allegheny to Oregon Avenues, is scheduled for completion in late 2022.

For more information about the waterfront, visit the Delaware River Waterfront Corporation's website at delawareriverwaterfront.com.

Walk Description

Start at the Residences at Dockside (717 S. Columbus Blvd.), a 16-story apartment building resembling a luxury ocean liner with "smokestacks" on top. *Open-Air Aquarium* features a school of steel fish swimming in the air.

Walk north along the Delaware. ❶ **Battleship *New Jersey,*** docked across the river in Camden, New Jersey, was launched in December 1942 and was directly involved in key Pacific battles during World War II. The ship was used during the Korean and Vietnam Wars, provided support during the Lebanese Civil War in the 1980s, and served troops during the First Gulf War. Today it's a museum and a memorial to its sailors.

At Lombard Circle, turn right, continuing along the water. ❷ *Moshulu,* now a floating restaurant and event venue, previously sailed under different flags. Built in Scotland in 1904, the vessel first carried coal from Germany to Chile, returning to Europe with nitrate. In more than a decade at sea, the ship successfully navigated Cape Horn 54 times.

During World War I, the US confiscated the ship while it was docked in an American port. President Woodrow Wilson's wife redubbed it *Moshulu,* a Seneca word meaning "one who fears nothing." *Moshulu* has occupied its current berth since 2002. Catch the ship in *Rocky,* as the fighter exercises along the waterfront, and in *The Godfather: Part II,* carrying the young Vito Corleone to America.

Across from *Moshulu,* a plaque honors citizen-soldiers who watched the waterfront in 1747. The group was a predecessor to the Pennsylvania National Guard.

Continue to the ❸ **USS *Becuna,*** a Connecticut-built submarine that patrolled the Pacific during World War II, sinking four enemy ships. The sub spied on Russian submarines during the Cold War and monitored the Mediterranean and Atlantic Oceans during the Korean and Vietnam Wars. Decommissioned in 1969, it's now a museum with guided tours provided by former sailors. One guide explained that subs were nicknamed pig boats, sharing this joke: A man wanted to bring live pigs aboard a submarine. A fellow sailor said, "But what about the smell?" The first man replied, "They'll get used to it. We all did."

Next to the sub is the warship USS *Olympia*. Launched in 1892, it's the only surviving vessel from the Spanish-American War fleet. Commodore George Dewey delivered the famous words, "You may fire when you are ready, Gridley," in 1898 on the Olympia's deck when American forces were fighting in Manila Bay. The ship's last mission, in 1921, was carrying the body of the unknown soldier from France to the United States. The neighboring World War II Submariners Memorial honors sailors on eternal patrol.

④ **Spruce Street Harbor Park** is a warm-weather pop-up park with free games, a beer garden and food, and hammocks. A cantilevered net lounge allows visitors to stretch out 4 feet above the water—with a second net below to catch fallen wallets and cell phones.

The Hope Fence, along the Hilton Philadelphia at Penn's Landing (201 S. Columbus Blvd.), is a 250-foot "love lock" fence that invites people to commemorate significant moments in their lives by attaching a lock. It was inspired by Paris's Ponts des Arts, where couples place padlocks bearing their names to the railing or grate, then toss the key into the Seine River.

The Ben Franklin Bridge links Philadelphia to Camden, New Jersey.

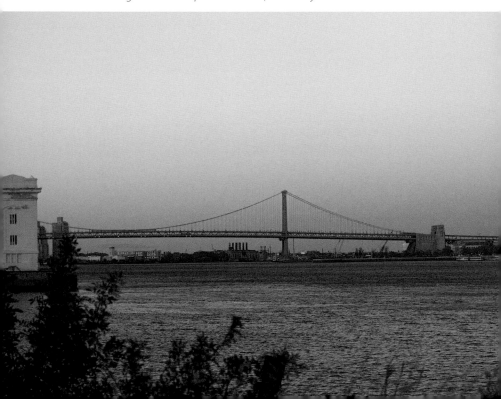

Gazela Primeiro, a 120-year-old wooden tall ship, has been moored on the Delaware River since 1971. Built in Portugal to carry cod fishermen to the Grand Banks of Newfoundland, the ship was used for commercial purposes until 1969. The nonprofit Philadelphia Ship Preservation Guild is rebuilding the ship using the same natural materials with which it was first constructed. *Gazela* had a role in 1984's *Interview with the Vampire:* Brad Pitt filmed scenes on her deck.

Continue along the river. The ❺ **Independence Seaport Museum** offers hands-on programming. A marker remembers the *Hughes Glomar Explorer,* a ship built in nearby Chester in the 1970s. Workers believed the boat was for billionaire Howard Hughes. In truth it was a CIA project designed to find a sunken Soviet submarine. The mission was successful. The bodies of six sailors were recovered and buried at sea.

Continue through Penn's Landing's Great Plaza, an open-air event space. Across the water, Camden City Hall is engraved with the Walt Whitman line, "In a dream I saw a city invincible." Camden is known for its political corruption scandals, with three mayors jailed in a 20-year period.

Pass ❻ **Blue Cross RiverRink,** which hosts Winterfest and Summerfest, both free events. Continue to the end of the pier, following it left to exit. At Columbus Boulevard, turn right and continue north.

❼ **Cherry Street Pier** (121 N. Columbus Blvd.), formerly known as Municipal Pier 9, is a mixed-use public space housed in a 55,000 square-foot former warehouse. Opened in 2018, Cherry Street offers resident artist studios in former shipping containers, food, a full bar, community event spaces, and an open-air garden framed by historic steel trusses. A pink vending machine here sells yarn and knitting needles.

❽ **Race Street Pier,** in the shadow of the Benjamin Franklin Bridge, is a multitiered park landscaped with 37 swamp white oak trees and more than 10,000 steel planters of sturdy grasses and perennials. The Delaware is a tidal river with fluctuating elevation, and the pier is one of the few places where visitors can get close to the water, guided by the pier's solar lights.

Across the street, ❾ **FringeArts** has a theater, a lauded French restaurant, and a gallery space in a former 1903 pumping station.

The ❿ **Benjamin Franklin Bridge,** connecting Philadelphia and Camden, was completed in 1926. On its first day of use, July 1, President Calvin Coolidge was on hand to dedicate the bridge, then the longest suspension bridge in the world. The concrete pier tower bears the Seal of Philadelphia. The bridge is lit to mark different occasions, becoming red, white, and blue on Pearl Harbor Day and welcoming the new year with a rainbow. In 2013's *World War Z,* military and police officers attempt to stop invading zombies on the bridge.

Morgan's Pier (221 N. Columbus Blvd.) is a warm-weather beer garden with food and live music. It's named for construction worker George Morgan, the first person to cross the Ben Franklin Bridge in the 1920s. Despite being told not to do so by a supervisor, Morgan reportedly crossed the final 50 feet of the incomplete footbridge by carefully balancing on a support cable 400 feet in the air. He was immediately fired.

Ahead is *Our Flag Unfurled* (500 N. Columbus Blvd.), originally painted after the 9/11 terrorist attacks. The mural was meant to be temporary but was refurbished for the 2016 Democratic National Convention.

At Callowhill Street, turn left. The street is named for William Penn's wife, Hannah Callowhill Penn. This was also called Gallows' Hill because it was the site of multiple public hangings. Hidden cityphila.org says this was Philadelphia's first red-light district: "Prostitutes frequented the sector's hostels and boarding houses, and pirates of the Atlantic Coast openly swaggered along Front and Callowhill Streets. Working and retired sea robbers, including Blackbeard and "Captain" William Kidd, liked Philadelphia because of the mild temper of Quaker Justice."

Continue on Callowhill Street. *History of Immigration* and *Freedom Wall* (Callowhill and N. Second Sts.) celebrate the city's diversity. The first panel shows Native Americans, ships afloat, and arriving immigrants, including Africans, Chinese, Europeans, and Central and South Americans. The second includes the Statue of Liberty and Martin Luther King Jr.

At North Seventh Street, turn left. ⑪ **Franklin Square** is one of the city's five original green spaces. After decades of neglect, the nonprofit Historic Philadelphia reclaimed the space in 2006, adding a carousel, two playgrounds, a minigolf course, and dining options.

Before exploring the square, cross to North Sixth Street. *City in Retrospect,* on the wall of the I-676 exit at Callowhill Street, depicts an old-fashioned street scene painted with black-and-white and sepia tones. *Electric Philadelphia,* a mural with neonlike LED lights, brightens the underpass.

Walk south on North Sixth Street to the 101-foot-tall silver steel sculpture *Bolt of Lightning,* which remembers Franklin's famous experiment. A key at the base is topped with a jagged bolt and hints of a kite. In 2010, a *Philadelphia* critic called it "the blunder at the bridge," quoting a bridge authority saying, "It's so damn ugly, it'll take people's minds off the higher tolls."

This walk ends here. To keep moving, continue three blocks south on Sixth Street to Independence Hall.

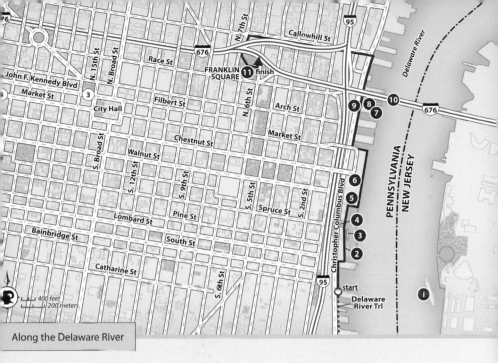

Along the Delaware River

Points of Interest

1. **Battleship *New Jersey*** 62 Battleship Place, 856-966-1652, battleshipnewjersey.org
2. ***Moshulu*** 401 S. Columbus Blvd., 215-923-2500, moshulu.com
3. **USS *Becuna*** S. Columbus Blvd. and Market St., 215-928-8807, delawareriverwaterfront.com
4. **Spruce Street Harbor Park** S. Columbus Blvd. and Spruce St., 215-922-2386, delawareriverwaterfront.com
5. **Independence Seaport Museum** 211 S. Columbus Blvd., 215-413-8655, phillyseaport.org
6. **Blue Cross RiverRink** 101 S. Columbus Blvd., 215-925-7465, delawareriverwaterfront.com
7. **Cherry Street Pier** 121 N. Columbus Blvd., 215-923-0818, cherrystreetpier.com
8. **Race Street Pier** Race St. and N. Columbus Blvd., 215-922-2386, delawareriverwaterfront.com
9. **FringeArts** 140 N. Columbus Blvd., 215-413-9006, fringearts.com
10. **Benjamin Franklin Bridge** 856-968-3300, drpa.org
11. **Franklin Square** 200 N. Sixth St., 215-629-4026, historicphiladelphia.org/franklin-square

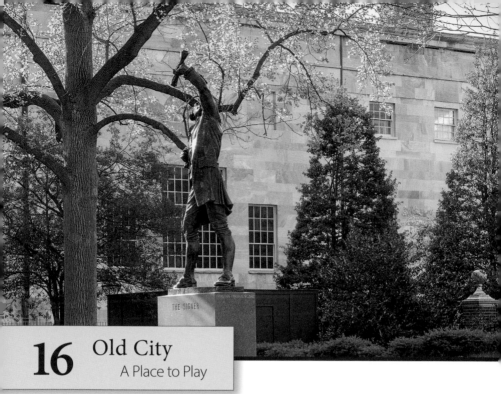

16 Old City
A Place to Play

THE SIGNER

Above: This statue in Signers Garden is a tribute to the daring men who committed the treasonous act of signing the Declaration of Independence.

BOUNDARIES: Vine St., Chestnut St., S. Fifth St., Front St.
DISTANCE: 1.9 miles
DIFFICULTY: Easy
PARKING: Street parking is challenging, but there is a 24-hour secured parking lot underneath the Independence Visitor Center.
PUBLIC TRANSIT: There is a SEPTA subway stop at Market and S. Fifth Sts.

Old City has been called Philadelphia's SoHo because of its boutiques, restaurants, nightclubs, studios, and galleries. Art galleries open their doors on the first Friday of every month, attracting hundreds of visitors.

This was the city's earliest commercial area—its tiny alleys used to transport goods by foot or cart from the Delaware River to points inland.

Many of the area's residential properties are condos or rental apartments in former industrial spaces. The marked exception is Elfreth's Alley, the nation's oldest residential street.

Walk Description

Begin on the southeast corner of South Sixth and Walnut Streets across from Washington Square. Walnut Street Prison, built in 1773, once sprawled over these blocks. In 1790, it became the nation's first penitentiary, so called because Quakers believed that, in the right environment, prisoners could reflect on their crimes and truly repent. One of the men who served time was Robert Morris, one of only six people who signed both the Declaration of Independence and the Constitution. The so-called financier of the Revolution, Morris was the second-most powerful man in the colonies after George Washington. Despite using his fortune to keep the country afloat during the Revolutionary War, Morris was jailed for three years for not paying debts. Washington visited him at Walnut Street Prison.

Cross Walnut Street. Enter Independence Park and take the path to the right of the sculpture in the center. Commodore John Barry, the "Father of the American Navy," is an oft overlooked hero of the American Revolution. A ship under his command was the first to capture a British war vessel at sea. Barry, nicknamed "Big John" because he was 6'4" and broad chested, is remembered as a fair, caring man at sea and on land. He was an early supporter of the Charitable Captains of Seas Club, which provided relief to families of lost sailors.

To exit, follow the path opposite the one you took to enter to South Fifth Street. Turn left. Benjamin Franklin founded the ❶ **American Philosophical Society** in 1743 to promote "useful knowledge," according to his memoirs. The organization is still active.

Continue to Signers Garden (500 Chestnut St.), a park honoring the men who risked their lives for the treasonous act of signing the Declaration of Independence. The center statue depicts Philadelphia-born George Clymer, another of the six to sign both of the country's founding documents.

Continue north on South Fifth Street. ❷ **The Philadelphia Bourse** originally housed a stock exchange, a maritime exchange, and a grain-trading center. The reddish-orange building, constructed in the 1890s, was inspired by a similar structure in Germany. The space now houses offices, shops, a movie theater, and a 30-vendor food court.

Next door, the ❸ **Weitzman National Museum of American Jewish History** was established in 1976 at nearby Congregation Mikveh Israel and moved here in 2010. Director Steven Spielberg's first 8 mm camera is on exhibit. The Only in America Gallery/Hall of Fame is free to enter. Among those featured is poet Emma Lazarus, whose most famous work includes, "Give me your tired, your poor, your huddled masses yearning to breathe free." The museum was closed for more than two years due to financial issues, reopening in 2022 with a sculpture by Deborah Kass in front: Large yellow letters reading OY/YO, depending on where the viewer stands, a shout out to Yiddish and Philadelphia-ese.

Cross Market Street, walking north. The mirror-polished steel sculpture *Gift of the Winds* (North Fifth and Market Sts.) evokes trees and leaves. The ❹ **Faith and Liberty Discovery Center** is run by the American Bible Society, which is headquartered here. Completed in May 2021, the attraction looks at how the Bible shaped the country's founding and its continued impact.

❺ **Congregation Mikveh Israel** stretches between North Fifth and North Fourth Streets, with its main doors at 44 N. Fourth St. It is the county's oldest continuously operating congregation and often called the "Synagogue of the American Revolution."

Arden Theatre Company sits in the heart of Old City.

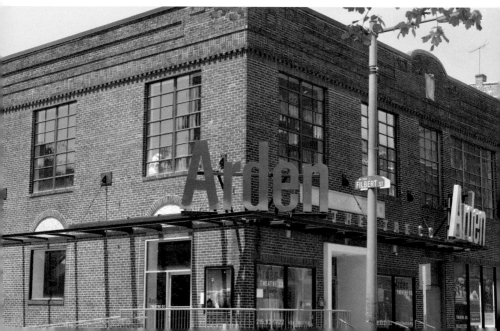

Follow the redbrick path at right. Pass the statue of Uriah P. Levy, the Navy's first Jewish commodore. Philadelphia-born Levy ran away at age 10 to be a ship's cabin boy, returning to celebrate his Bar Mitzvah at Mikveh Israel. Years later, he purchased Thomas Jefferson's Monticello, opening it to tourists.

Ahead are four white granite blocks in a square formation, a memorial to Jonathan Netanyahu, brother of Israeli prime minister Benjamin Netanyahu. Jonathan Netanyahu was an Israeli special forces officer killed while attempting to rescue 106 hostages taken during a plane hijacking. The Netanyahu family lived in Philadelphia while the patriarch taught here. At the 1986 memorial dedication, Benjamin said the family's Philadelphia years were a "pivotal passage point" for Jonathan, when "much of his character was formed. Month by month, he grew to appreciate the values of American life—openness, freedom, democracy. Those values stayed with him."

At North Fourth Street, turn right. A marker remembers congregant Haym Salomon, another Revolutionary War financier who was never repaid and died penniless. In 1975, a commemorative stamp honoring Salomon called him a "financial hero . . . responsible for raising most of the money needed to finance the American Revolution and later to save the new nation from collapse."

At Market Street, turn left. At North Third Street, turn left. This stretch of road has another name: N3rd, pronounced "nerd." It acknowledges the dozens of tech and design companies settling here.

Pass Harry's Smoke Shop (14 N. Third St.), which has been in business since 1938.

Continue north. The Tuttleman Brothers and Fagen building (56–60 N. Second St.) was a clothing manufacturer, renovated in 1900 with one of the country's last cast iron facades. It was one of the first neighborhood buildings converted to lofts.

❻ The Center for Art in Wood is a nonprofit supporting wood arts. Its mural highlights 100 objects in the museum's collection.

Cross Race Street. Wireworks (301 Race St.) is a former insulated-wire manufacturing business converted to condos in the 1980s. The English immigrant who founded the company originally made wire for bonnets and hoop skirts, then began producing copper wire, supplying all that Samuel Morse needed in 1844 for the first telegraph from Washington to Baltimore.

Pass beneath the Benjamin Franklin Bridge. The Chocolate Works (231 N. Third St.) is a residential rental complex in the former H. O. Wilbur & Sons Chocolate Company. Wilbur and a partner started their company in 1865, making molasses and hard candies that train boys sold to passengers.

❼ *Growth of a Metropolis* showcases Philadelphia architecture from 1682 to 2015. It wraps around the building; walk through the parking lot to see the second wall. The main wall features well-known structures, including City Hall. The side wall features three William Rush sculptures on display at the Philadelphia Museum of Art.

Continue on North Third Street, passing the former K. Strauss & Co., a cigar and cigarette manufacturing building, now condominiums. Thomas Scientific, at Vine and N. Third Streets, produces lab products on land once owned by Betsy Ross's father.

Turn left on Vine Street, then left again on North Fourth Street. **8** **St. Augustine Church,** founded in 1796, was the Augustinian Order's first permanent establishment in the United States. The church school, St. Augustine Academy for Boys, moved to the suburbs and became Villanova University. The exterior is in the films *The Sixth Sense* and *Shooter*. Today's congregation is largely Filipino. The choir sings songs in Tagalog and honors Santo Nino, the patron saint of the Philippines, each August.

Across the street, **9** **Historic St. George's United Methodist Church** is the cradle of American Methodism, in continuous use by Methodists since 1769. In the 1700s, the church welcomed African American worshippers to a special weekly service—held at 5 a.m. This upset two parishioners: Richard Allen, who left to found Mother Bethel African Methodist Episcopal Church, and Absalom Jones, who created the African Protestant Episcopal Church. In December 1776, war financier Robert Morris prayed all night here as he sought guidance on securing money for Washington's troops. In 1777, British soldiers occupying the city used the church as a cavalry school because it had a street-level door.

Continue south. Old First Reformed United Church of Christ (151 N. Fourth St.) was founded in the 1700s by German immigrants and used as a hospital by the British during the Revolution.

Turn left on Race Street. The Brass Works condominium building (231 Race St.) housed Homer Brassworks, manufacturers of beer and ale pumps in the early 1800s. The circa 1885 Pfeiffer House (222–226 Race St.) made coal-transport buckets.

Continue on Race Street. **10** **Paddy's Pub Old City** is the nominal bar from TV's *It's Always Sunny in Philadelphia*.

At North Second Street, turn right. Elizabeth Drinker, who lived on this block, kept a detailed journal from 1758 to 1807. The 2,100-page diary was published in 1889 and gives insight into the lives of every day Philadelphians. A peace-loving Quaker, Drinker and her husband, Henry, remained neutral during the American Revolution, which resulted in Henry's arrest for treason. When the British occupied Philadelphia in 1780, soldiers took two of the Drinkers' horses despite Elizabeth's protests. When the British surrendered in 1781, celebrating citizens, angry about the Quakers' lack of support, attacked Quaker homes. The Drinkers' home had 70 glass panes broken.

The Fireman's Hall Museum (147–49 N. Second St.), housed in a 1902 firehouse, traces the history of firefighting in Philadelphia.

Continue to ⓫ **Elfreth's Alley,** the oldest continuously inhabited residential block in the country, with homes built between 1720 and 1830. Two adjacent houses, built in 1755, are now a public museum. In the 1800s, eight families—a total of 27 people—shared these two dwellings.

Continue on North Second Street. ⓬ **Arden Theatre Company,** founded in 1988, offers classes and educational programs, in addition to performances of traditional shows.

⓭ **Christ Church,** established in 1695, is sometimes called The Nation's Church. Notable early worshippers included George Washington and John Adams. Until the 2020 pandemic, the pastor had boasted that the church had hosted a Sunday service every weekend for more than 300 years.

Continue south, crossing Market Street and passing multiple late-night venues.

At Chestnut Street, turn left. ⓮ **The Plough & the Stars** is an Irish pub whose name references the banner carried by Irish citizens who revolted against the British in the 1916 Easter Rebellion. The pub is in the former Corn Exchange National Bank, built in 1903.

⓯ **Han Dynasty** is a Chinese restaurant known for its super-spicy food and super-cranky owner. (Some even call the restaurant Handy Nasty.) A 2013 *Philadelphia* article described owner Han Chiang thusly: "He's famous for cursing at customers. For exploding in the middle of his own dining rooms over perceived breaches in good taste or decorum and refusing to serve people who do something stupid—like asking for Americanized Chinese dishes that exist on his menus but that he thinks no one but children should order. If you don't know him for his restaurants or his food, you likely know him for the legend that has grown up around him. 'Oh, that guy that screams at people who order sweet-and-sour chicken . . . that's Han.'" Still, the food is worth the abuse.

This walk ends here. The South Philadelphia II tour (page 158) begins a few steps away.

Points of Interest

① **American Philosophical Society** 104 S. Fifth St., 215-440-3400, amphilsoc.org

② **Philadelphia Bourse/The Bourse** 111 S. Independence Mall E., 215-625-0300, tinyurl.com/philadelphiabourse

③ **Weitzman National Museum of American Jewish History** 101 S. Independence Mall E., 215-923-3811, theweitzman.org

④ **Faith and Liberty Discovery Center** 101 N. Independence Mall E, 215-309-0401, faithandliberty.org

⑤ **Congregation Mikveh Israel** 44 N. Fourth St., 215-922-5446, mikvehisrael.org

(continued on next page)

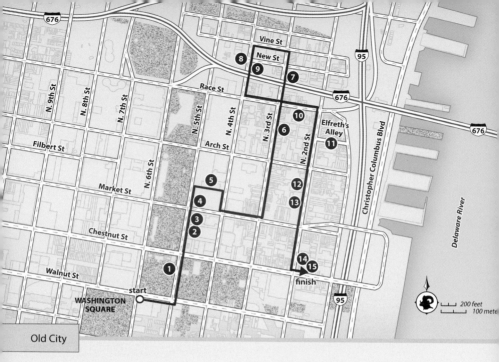

Old City

(continued from previous page)

6 **The Center for Art in Wood** 141 N. Third St., 215-923-8000, centerforartinwood.org

7 *Growth of a Metropolis* 251 N. Third St. Mural Arts Philadelphia, 215-685-0750, muralarts.org.

8 **St. Augustine Church** 243 N. Lawrence St., 215-627-1838, st-augustinechurch.com

9 **Historic St. George's United Methodist Church** 235 N. Fourth St., 215-925-7788, historicstgeorges.org

10 **Paddy's Pub Old City** 228 Race St., 215-627-3532, paddyspuboldcity.com

11 **Elfreth's Alley** Off N. Second St. between Arch and Race Sts., 215-627-8680 (museum house), elfrethsalley.org

12 **Arden Theatre Company** 40 N. Second St., 215-922-1122, ardentheatre.org

13 **Christ Church** 20 N. American St., 215-922-1695, christchurchphila.org

14 **The Plough & the Stars** 123 Chestnut St., 215-733-0300, ploughstars.com

15 **Han Dynasty** 123 Chestnut St., 215-922-1888, handynasty.net/oldcity

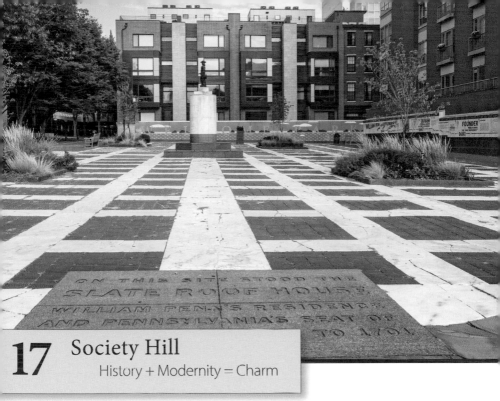

17 Society Hill
History + Modernity = Charm

BOUNDARIES: Dock St., S. Fourth St., Chestnut St., Lombard St.
DISTANCE: 2.1 miles
DIFFICULTY: Easy
PARKING: There are multiple paid garages but only a few metered street parking spots.
PUBLIC TRANSIT: Via subway, take the Market-Frankford line to Second Street Station. The buses that stop within a quarter mile are 12, 21, 25, 40, 42, and 57.

Settled in 1682, Society Hill is one of the city's oldest neighborhoods, named for the Free Society of Traders, which had offices here in the 1700s. Immediately before and after the Revolutionary War, the area flourished because of its location between the seat of government and the Delaware River.

Society Hill was neglected as the city expanded west. By 1940, it was completely run-down. City planner Edmund Bacon led the revitalization drive, which included purchasing 31 acres around Dock Street and hiring famed architect I. M. Pei to design residences there. Shabby homes were sold to buyers who promised to restore them. The city added brick sidewalks and replicas of 18th-century street lighting. Today this is one of the city's safest and wealthiest neighborhoods, with the country's largest collection of Georgian- and Federal-style brick row houses.

Walk Description

Begin at ① **Old Original Bookbinder's.** Founded in 1898 by Dutch Jewish immigrants, it was a popular fine dining spot famous for its lobster dishes and Bookbinder's Soup, a tomato-based stew made with snapping turtle and vegetables. Regular Frank Sinatra called the place Bookies. The exterior includes a plaque of Abraham Lincoln and the complete Gettysburg Address. It's now called The Olde Bar and operated by *Iron Chef* winner Jose Garces.

Walk west toward South Second Street. ② **City Tavern** is a replica of the original 1773 building where Thomas Jefferson reportedly ate most of his meals and John Jay rented a room. In 1773, Paul Revere rushed here with news of the Boston Tea Party. John Adams called this the "most genteel tavern in America." Two ghosts haunt the grounds: a woman killed in a fire as she prepared for her wedding and a waiter slain in a duel. The female ghost appears in photos. The male likes knocking down silverware. The modern restaurant closed in 2020.

At South Second Street, turn right. Welcome Park, between Walnut and Chestnut Streets, is the only city park dedicated to founder William Penn, whose home stood here. The park is named for the *Welcome,* the 17th-century ship that carried Penn from England. The surrounding walls are engraved with his city plans. Its original street grid is imprinted on the ground. The Penn statue is a miniature of the one atop City Hall.

To promote his new city, Penn prepared marketing materials saying it offered "seven ordinaries [taverns] for the entertainment of strangers . . . and a good meal is to be had for sixpence," according to Jim Murphy, author of *Real Philly History, Real Fast.*

Continue on South Second Street to Chestnut Street. The Corn Exchange National Bank (123–25 Chestnut St.) was built in 1903 in the Georgian Revival style. Bank robber Willie Sutton attempted to rob this bank in 1933 but failed. He and two partners returned a year later, leaving with more than $21,000.

Turn left. The 17-story ③ **U.S. Custom House** occupies an entire block. The interior features a three-story rotunda and elaborate murals.

Continue to South Third Street. Turn left. At left is the ④ **Museum of the American Revolution,** with exhibits including George Washington's war tent, a 1770s mug that smells of rum, and booties made from a Redcoat's jacket.

At right is part of Independence National Park. Outlined on the ground near the fence are the buildings that once stood here, including the Treasury Secretary Alexander Hamilton's office.

The **5** **First Bank of the United States** was chartered in 1791 and authorized by Congress to hold $10 million in capital. Hamilton lobbied for the bank's founding, saying it would be "a political machine of greatest importance to the state." His ghost reportedly haunts the structure.

Continue south to Walnut Street. At left is **6** **Merchants' Exchange Building,** the country's oldest existing stock exchange building. Opened in the 1830s, it was the hub of American commercial life for 50 years. The stunning Greek Revival building prompted one newspaper to write that "Philadelphia is truly the Athens of America."

Turn right onto Walnut Street. Ahead at 306 Walnut Street was the first branch of the Philadelphia Savings Fund Society. Founded in 1816, PSFS introduced a new type of bank, one in which depositors owned the bank's wealth. The façade's white marble was mined in nearby Chester County.

Next door, the Polish American Cultural Center (308 Walnut St.) includes a free museum featuring Thaddeus Kosciuszko, who played a crucial part in the patriots' Revolutionary War victory, and Casimir Pulaski, the so-called "Father of the American Cavalry."

Continue west. The **7** **Bishop White House** is reportedly one of the city's most haunted structures. This was the home of the Right Reverend William White, rector of Christ Church and first bishop of the American Episcopalian Church. During 1793's yellow fever epidemic, White tended the sick but stayed healthy, possibly because his constant cigar smoking kept mosquitoes away. He died in his third-floor library in 1836. His ghost is still seen there. A housekeeper haunts the first floor, and a ghost cat has been heard meowing in the garden.

Pass the Dilworth-Todd-Moylan House (339–41 Walnut St.), the former residence of Dolley Payne Todd, who married future president James Madison. Aaron Burr introduced the couple.

At South Fourth Street, turn left. **8** **The Philadelphia Contributionship** is the country's oldest property insurance company, organized by Ben Franklin in 1752. Homeowners who purchased fire protection were given fire marks to display on their property exterior. This told firefighters that they would be paid for their work by a specific insurer. The Contributionship created the colonies' first fire mark, which showed four hands, each holding the wrist of another, forming a box shape.

Continue on South Fourth, passing Bingham Court, a collection of homes between South Third and Fourth Streets, Willings Alley, and Spruce Street. The homes were designed by celebrated modernist architect I. M. Pei, whose work includes the Louvre Pyramid in Paris. It's named for William Bingham, a delegate to the Continental Congress and a US senator.

9 **Old St. Mary's Church,** built in 1763, was the city's second Roman Catholic church. Although none of the Founding Fathers were Catholic, they gathered here for the first public religious commemoration of the Declaration of Independence. Notables resting in the church cemetery include Commodore John Barry, Father of the American Navy, and George Meade, whose grandson would lead Union forces at Gettysburg.

Continue on South Fourth. **10** **Physick House** is the former home of Dr. Philip Syng Physick, the "Father of American Surgery." Physick's patients included President Andrew Jackson, Chief Justice John Marshall, and Dolley Madison. Displayed inside are Physick's tools, including blood-letting instruments, stomach pumps, and kidney stone removal tubes. The ghost of Physick's estranged wife haunts the property, crying outside.

Turn right on Cypress Street. This enclave, called Lawrence Court, was once home to 1976 Nobel Prize for Medicine winner Baruch Blumbert, who with colleagues discovered the hepatitis B virus and created its vaccine.

At the intersection of Cypress and Lawrence Court stand Harold Kimmelman's *Kangaroos*. A 2015 *Philadelphia* article included *Kangaroos* on a "12 Worst Pieces of Public Art" list. "Why? Why kangaroos? Why kangaroos here?" the author moaned.

Turn right on Lawrence Court. At Spruce Street, turn left. Society Hill Synagogue (418 Spruce St.) was originally a Baptist church. Jews from Romania purchased the building in 1912, and the Yiddish words "Great roumanian Shul" are above the door. The synagogue remains active.

The Museum of the American Revolution bears a relief of Washington crossing the Delaware.

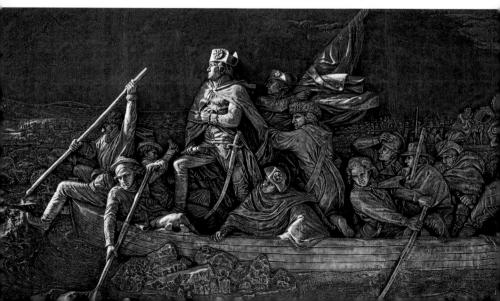

Across the road is the Coca-Cola Bottle House (433 Spruce St.). Built in 1972 for the CEO of the Coca-Cola Company, its two lower windows are made from soda bottles.

Continue west on Spruce Street, crossing South Fifth Street. Many of these private homes have long histories. In 1795, the home at 507 was built for comb maker John Fininister; his neighbor at 509, Schoolmaster Daniel Britt, settled there in 1797. The property at 519–21 belonged to engraver John Vallance in 1796. A historic marker notes that Vallance's name was on early bank notes. When Vallance's home was for sale in 2015 for $1 million, PhillyVoice.com noted Vallance's ties to early money were appropriate, as "you'd have to hand over a lot of bank notes to live here."

Continue, passing the former Rebecca Gratz Club (532 Spruce St.). The "club" was a boarding house for single Jewish women founded in the 1920s. It was named for Gratz, a 19th-century philanthropist who opened the first Jewish Sunday School and founded the Hebrew Women's Benevolent Society. The building is now apartments.

At South Sixth Street, turn right, with Washington Square Park at left. Make a right on the pedestrian alley at Locust Street, then cross South Fifth Street to reach St. Mary's Interparochial School (500 Locust St.). Like many city schools, St. Mary's doesn't have an adjoining playground. Instead, recess is held on the roof. Some schools have domed tops resembling fencing to keep balls from flying away.

St. Mary's students also play in the two nearby National Park Service–maintained public gardens. The Rose Garden is on the north side of Locust Street and the Magnolia Garden is on the south side. Thomas Jefferson wrote that "of all the countries in the world, America is where the noblest gardens may be made without expense."

Continue to South Fourth Street and turn left. At Willings Alley, turn right. ⓫ **Old St. Joseph's Church** is the city's first Roman Catholic parish, founded in 1733. At one point this was the only place in the English speaking world where Catholics could celebrate Mass publicly. The church's odd location—requiring entrance through the small alley archway—was chosen to dissuade protesters. Still, the building suffered damage during anti-Catholic riots in the 1800s.

At the alley's end, look left. Thomas Paine's *Common Sense* pamphlet, printed on Thomas Paine Place, in January 1776, played a crucial part in galvanizing colonists against England by laying out arguments in simple language. He referred to King George as "a crowned ruffian" with "little more to do than make war and give away places at court."

Ahead is St. Paul's Episcopal Church (225 S. Third St.), built in 1761. Acclaimed American actor Edwin Forrest is interred in its graveyard.

The two-story building at right occupies land with a rich, now unseen, history. In 2017, Hidden City Philadelphia said that it would be difficult to find a location with "more lost built history" than this one, which is "indicative of Philadelphia's unyielding habit of demolition for redevelopment." The Willing family mansion was the first structure on the lot, built in 1745. In the 1830s, Dr. Thomas Dent Mutter had his offices here. In the 1850s, the Pennsylvania Railroad Company razed the mansion and built a new headquarters here. In the years that followed, this land held a gas station and a playground. Dr. Roshen Irani built this Postmodernist building as her home in the 1970s and left it to St. Joseph's Church when she died in 2007.

Turn right, walking south on South Third Street. ⑫ **The Powel House,** built in 1765, was the home of Samuel Powel, the city's last Colonial and first post-Revolutionary War mayor. While Samuel, a pallbearer at Benjamin Franklin's funeral, is remembered as the family's politician, it was his wife, Elizabeth, who advised George Washington on personal and state matters. The Washingtons frequently dined here and later hosted the Powels at Mount Vernon.

The Powels' neighbor, at 242 S. Third Street, was Juan de Miralles, a Spanish diplomat who funneled financial assistance from Spain to the upstart colonials.

Continue to Pine Street. The ⑬ **Thaddeus Kosciuszko National Memorial** is a single room where the Polish-born Kosciuszko lived for seven months. NPR's 2008 piece titled "The Smallest National Park Site," notes "It's an inspiration to renters everywhere that a cheap studio apartment could become part of the National Park System." Kosciuszko was a brigadier general during the Revolutionary War, using his engineering background to construct state-of-the-art defenses at various fortifications. Thomas Jefferson called him "the purest son of liberty I have ever known."

At Pine Street, turn right. ⑭ **St. Peter's Church** opened in 1758 to handle overflow from nearby Christ Church. The interior maintains its "boxed pews," individual cubes with seating on three sides accessed by a small door on the fourth. Worshippers reserved boxes as late as 1966. The current rector, Claire Nevin-Field, is the first female leader in the church's history. The church's first leader, Reverend William White, looks staid in paintings, but Nevin-Field called him "a wild man in his day." One of his bold acts? Ordaining the Episcopal Church's first African American priest.

Continue west, crossing South Fourth Street. ⑮ **Old Pine Street Church** was used as a stable by the British cavalry when they occupied the city during the Revolutionary War. The adjoining cemetery, opened in 1764, holds an estimated 3,000 people. The last person buried here, in 1958, was University of Pennsylvania student In-Ho Oh, a Korean native fatally beaten by teenagers seeking cash to buy 65-cent dance tickets. Oh's tombstone contains the words, "To turn sorrow into a Christian purpose." In 2016, Philadelphia Councilperson David Oh, In-Ho Oh's cousin, successfully led efforts to have the West Philadelphia block where Oh was killed named in his honor.

In Old Pine Street Church's cemetery, note the likeness of Reverend George Duffield hand-chiseled onto a 16-foot-tall maple tree stump. Duffield, co-chaplain of the Continental

Army, was an inspiring speaker whose sermons convinced John Adams to sign the Declaration of Independence.

At South Fifth Street, turn left. At Lombard Street, turn left again. The ⓖ **Presbyterian Historical Society,** organized in 1852, contains the Presbyterian Church's national archives. Six 9-foot-tall statues by Alexander Stirling Calder depict Presbyterian leaders, including John Witherspoon, the only clergy member to sign the Declaration of Independence, and James Caldwell, the so-called "Fighting Parson," who, when troops ran out of gun wadding during the Revolutionary War, passed out pages from psalm books.

Continue east. The Old Pine Community Center (401 Pine St.) is a nonprofit community hub with programs including 12-step meetings, wheelchair basketball games, after-school care, and senior activities.

At South Fourth Street, cross the road, then turn left. St. Peter's Episcopal Churchyard is the final resting place of notable politicians, doctors, and military leaders, including artist Charles Willson Peale, who painted more than 1,000 portraits of Revolutionary War leaders and prominent citizens. It also holds the remains of eight Native American tribal leaders who caught small pox when they came to Philadelphia in January 1793 to discuss boundaries with President Washington. Their graves are not marked.

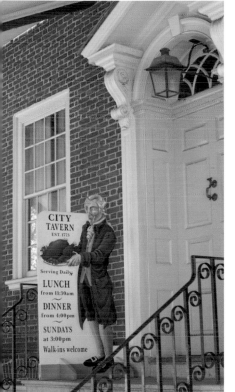

City Tavern, rebuilt at this spot, was popular with the Founding Fathers.

Continue on South Fourth Street. At Delancey Street, turn right. Pass Delancey Park, known locally as *Three Bears* because of the sculpture added in 1966. Take note of the Philadelphia Contributionship's fire marks on 318 and 320 Delancey Street. The fire mark at 300 Delancey Street is a tree. These were issued by Mutual Assurance of Philadelphia, aka The Green Tree Company, in the 1820s. Its symbol acknowledges it insured properties near trees, which others did not.

Cross South Third Street. Historic touches include horse-head hitching posts and boot scrapers near many front steps. A more modern addition? Electric vehicle parking and charging stations between 214 and 216. *Butterfly* (210 Delancey St.) is by kangaroo-loving sculptor Kimmelman.

At South Second Street, turn left. At Spruce Street, the shuttered building on the right was **⓱ A Man Full of Trouble Tavern,** built in 1759, the only surviving tavern from pre-Revolutionary Philadelphia. Taverns were central to 16th-century social life; one survey from 1773 tallied 120 in the city, with 21 on South Second Street alone. Historians say this tavern was originally called The Man Loaded with Mischief. Its sign featured a man carrying a woman on his back.

Continue north. The property at 210 S. Second Street was built for the family of British Navy Captain James Abercrombie in 1756. His son, also named James, became pastor at St. Peter's Episcopal Church in 1794. After noticing that President George Washington would leave the church before receiving communion, Abercrombie gave a sermon chastising those who did not do so. It was aimed at Washington, and the president knew it, but he did not change his practices. Historian Paul Boller suggests Washington did not want to be a hypocrite, taking communion after promoting, fighting, and winning a bloody war.

Continue straight. **⓲ Society Hill Towers**, three 31-story high-rises, were also designed by I. M. Pei. The style is brutalist, which also describes the featured sculpture. *Old Man, Young Man, the Future* shows a young man standing, an older man sitting, and a bird. Sculptor Leonard Baskin was known for work dealing with "the human-condition in angst-ridden terms. . . . If his figures did not appear to be actively suffering or simply dead, they often appeared to be in numbed, introspective states," noted 2003's *I. M. Pei and Society Hill: A 40th Anniversary Celebration*. Baskin said the bird represents the future and the "promising and ominous" nature of external reality.

At Locust Street, turn left. Pei wanted to create 37 contemporary brick-and-glass houses that were "sympathetic with the old 18th-century houses, but obviously they had to be designed around contemporary life" and cheap to build. The boxlike exteriors belie the light and airy interiors.

This tour ends here. Pick up Walk 15 (page 92) by turning around and following Spruce Street to the Delaware River.

Points of Interest

① **Old Original Bookbinder's (now The Olde Bar)** 125 Walnut St., 215-253-3777, theoldebar.com

② **City Tavern** 138 S. Second St., 215-413-1443, citytavern.com

③ **U.S. Custom House** 200 Chestnut St., gsa.gov/historic-buildings/us-custom-house-philadelphia-pa

④ **Museum of the American Revolution** 101 S. Third St., 215-253-6731, amrevmuseum.org

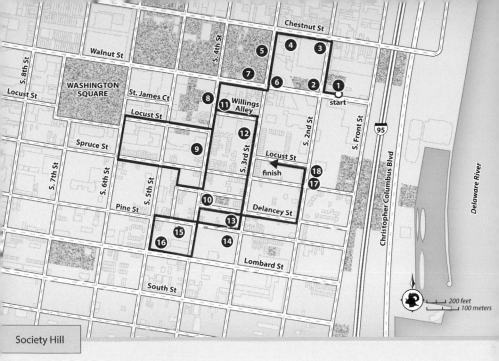

⑤ First Bank of the United States 116 S. Third St., 215-965-2305, nps.gov/inde

⑥ Merchants' Exchange Building 143 S. Third St., 215-965-2305, nps.gov/inde

⑦ Bishop White House 309 Walnut St., 215-965-2305, nps.gov/inde

⑧ The Philadelphia Contributionship 210 S. Fourth St., contributionship.com

⑨ Old St. Mary's Church 252 S. Fourth St., 215-923-7930, oldstmary.com

⑩ Physick House 321 S. Fourth St., 215-925-7866, philalandmarks.org/physick-house

⑪ Old St. Joseph's Church 321 Willings Alley, 215-923-1733, oldstjoseph.org

⑫ The Powel House 244 S. Third St., 215-627-0364, philalandmarks.org/powel-house

⑬ Thaddeus Kosciuszko National Memorial 301 Pine St., 215-597-8787, nps.gov/thko

⑭ St. Peter's Church 313 Pine St., 215-925-5968, stpetersphila.org

⑮ Old Pine Street Church 412 Pine St., 215-925-8051, oldpine.org

⑯ Presbyterian Historical Society 425 Lombard St., 215-627-1852, history.pcusa.org

⑰ A Man Full of Trouble Tavern 125 Spruce St.

⑱ Society Hill Towers 200–220 Locust St.

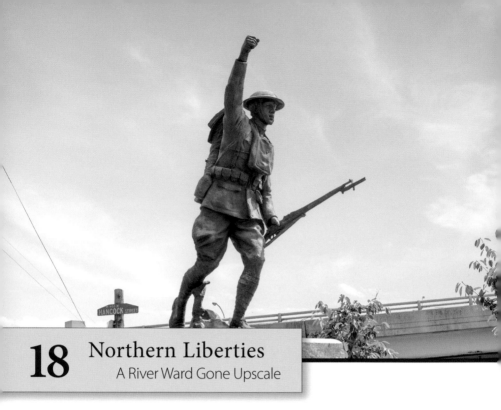

18 Northern Liberties
A River Ward Gone Upscale

Above: Doughboy Park in Northern Liberties honors World War I service members.

BOUNDARIES: Spring Garden St., Girard Ave., N. Second St., N. Eighth St.
DISTANCE: 3.5 miles
DIFFICULTY: Moderate
PARKING: It's usually fairly easy to find street parking here; there are also paid lots nearby.
PUBLIC TRANSIT: The Spring Garden subway station is located at 600 N. Front St. Area buses include the 43.

In 2014, a museum hosted a lecture called "Northern Liberties: From the World's Workshop to Hipster Mecca and the People in Between." That's one way to describe how this former industrial neighborhood has changed, but it's not the whole story.

One of Philadelphia's river wards, the area was outside city limits when William Penn founded Philadelphia. Called the north lands, it was part of the liberties, free land parcels granted at government discretion. The area was densely populated in the 1800s, with men, women, and children working mills and factories that produced everything from chocolate to machinery. When industry floundered, so did the neighborhood. Between 1960 and 1980, more than 60% of the population left. Blight followed. Its fortune began to change in the 1990s. Expect construction on this tour.

Walk Description

Start at North Second and Spring Garden Streets. ❶ *Pedal Thru (Bikin' in the O-Zone)* wraps around City Fitness, showing a bicycle moving through a city. The mural is visible to drivers stuck in traffic on nearby I-95.

Cross Spring Garden Street to ❷ **Doughboy Park.** Dedicated in 1920 to local World War I servicemen, this triangle features greenery, benches, cobblestones, and the bronze soldier statue, *Over the Top,* by John Paulding.

Walk north on North Second Street. This street was laid out in the 1700s and paved in 1761. The area is known for its nightlife, a reputation gained in its earliest days. No police patrolled here until the neighborhood joined the city in the mid 1850s, and the area "has had a history of rioting and disorder—as well as drunkenness and decadence—going back three hundred years," writes Harry Kyriakodis in *Northern Liberties: The Story of a Philadelphia River Ward.*

The building at 621–623 was an ornamental cast iron factory before being converted to condos in 2005. Architectural Antiques Exchange (721 N. Second St.) has three floors of inventory that includes century-old bars, vintage furniture, and antique fireplace mantels.

Continue for two blocks. The building at 901 has housed pubs for more than 200 years. The current one, ❸ **Standard Tap,** dates to 1999. Philly is known for its gastropubs, and this is considered the first. Two ghosts allegedly haunt the structure, a white-haired woman, who just stands around, and a former male tenant, who turns on water faucets and empties paper towel holders.

Continue on North Second. ❹ **North Bowl** was a mechanic's garage converted in 2006 to a retro-chic bowling alley with a full bar and music. The website Thrillist.com included it on its 2013 list of "The Swankiest, Tastiest, Booziest Bowling Alleys in America."

Cescaphe Ballroom, an event space at 935 N. Second St., stands where the Imperial Theater presented first silent movies, then talkies, for more than 30 years beginning in 1923. Before that it was the Bull's Head Tavern and Hotel. In 1809, "the staid citizens of Philadelphia were agog with curiosity over a strange and mysterious thing upon a vacant tract beside the Bull's Head Tavern," according to the Library Company of Philadelphia. They were looking at plans for the country's first railroad.

At West Laurel Street, turn right. At Hancock Street, go left. Many of these factories, now apartments and condos, operated in the years before child labor laws. *A Guide to Northern Liberties,* published in 1982 by the Northern Liberties Neighborhood Association, mentions a weaving mill that in 1832 employed 114 men and women. The men averaged $8.50 per week, and the women, $2.62. The children received $1.37.

The building at 1010 N. Hancock Street was once part of Schmidt & Sons Brewery, prompting one new business tenant to write "Cheers" on the wall behind its reception desk. The Carriage House Lofts (1011 N. Hancock St.) were built in the 1700s and once produced hubs and spokes for carriage wheels.

Continue to *Bebot,* a 33-foot-tall, 13,000-pound robot sculpture originally seen at the 2018 Burning Man Festival, which stands at an entrance to ❺ **The Piazza,** a mixed-use development located where the aforementioned Schmidt's Brewery operated from 1860 to 1987. At its mid-1970s peak, the brewery was producing more than 4 million barrels of beer annually.

Walk through the Piazza, exiting on North Second Street. Turn left. At Laurel Street, turn right. Ahead is ❻ **Liberty Lands Park,** which occupies the former Burks Brothers Tannery and Leather Factory, once the world's second-largest kid glove manufacturer.

Circle the park, turning right on Bodine St, passing the community garden, turning left on Wildey Street, then left again on North Third Street.

At the park entrance, Dennis Haugh's *Cohocksink: Stand in the Place Where You Live,* remembers the Delaware River subsidiary, now filled in, that periodically swallowed people and property. After an 1894 storm, phillyhistory.org notes, there was a "familiar 'deep rumbling' heard throughout Northern Liberties. Everyone knew what happened: the Cohocksink claimed yet another chunk of the city."

Continue on North Third Street. Pass the century-old Kaplan's New Model Bakery (901 N. Third St.) and Ortlieb's (847 N. Third St.), a music venue occupying the former company store of the Henry F. Ortlieb Brewing Company.

Thomas Mifflin School (808 N. Third St.), built in 1825, was used as a hospital during the 1832 cholera outbreak. The Northern Liberties Neighborhood Association (700 N. Third St.) opened The Yard, its new public park, in 2018.

At Fairmount Avenue, turn right. *Advocates for Advocacy* (306 Fairmount Ave.) is by acclaimed street artist Brett Cook-Dizney. The Zimmerman Building (425 Fairmount Ave.) was originally a slaughterhouse. Note the life-size terra-cotta bull's heads in the cornice.

❼ **Saint Michael the Archangel Orthodox Church** was built in 1873 for the Salem German Reform Church. The current congregation, many of Russian, Galician, and Carpatho-Russian

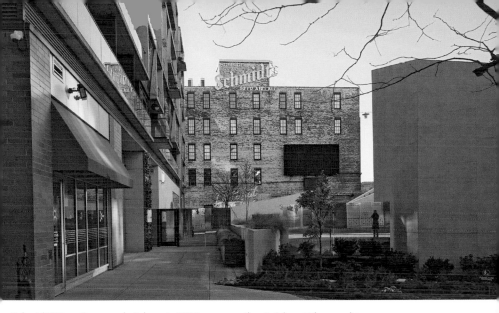

Schmidt & Sons Brewery, shut down in 1987, was once the city's largest beer maker.

heritage, purchased it in 1923. The church shop sells Russian goods, including *matryoshka* dolls, and it has hosted an annual Russian Festival for more than 40 years.

At North Fifth Street, turn right. **8** **Saint Andrew's Russian Orthodox Cathedral,** established in 1897, is the city's oldest Orthodox Christian church. It exists thanks to Russian Imperial Fleet representatives who came to the city in 1898 to help build two battleships, then gave time, money, and icons to the new church. The cathedral was consecrated in 1902 by Father Alexander Hotovitzky, who later died under Stalin's rule.

Through Cracks in Pavement (717 N. Fifth St.) features medicinal plants, flowers, barks, leaves, and roots. Artist Paul Santoleri was inspired by his brick-paved backyard, according to philaplace. org. He included a columbine to "reclaim the flower from the news of past years."

Turn right on Olive Street. At North Fourth Street, turn left. At Brown Street, look right. St. Agnes–St. John Nepomucene (Slovak), at 319 Brown Street, is two churches that merged in 1980 at the St. Agnes property.

Turn left on Brown Street. The African Zoar Episcopal Church was founded on this corner in 1794 by African Americans seeking a safe worship place. The Hebrew word "Zoar" means "good-will." A stop on the Underground Railroad, the church was the meeting place for the neighborhood "Vigilance Committee" in the 1830s. The committee said its role was to protect free blacks from kidnapping, but it actually assisted those escaping slavery.

Continue to North Fifth Street. The GA Bislar Paper Box Company (729 N. Fifth St.) was the country's largest producer of paper boxes in the 19th century, employing 1,900 people and making packaging for everything from hosiery to candy. It's now Liberties Lofts.

Turn right on North Fifth Street. Parts of this stretch feel different from other parts of the neighborhood. At Poplar Street, turn right. *Philos Adelphos* (440 Poplar St.) is by Mexican artist Saner Edgar.

Turn around and make a diagonal right on St. John Neumann Way, wrapping around Bardot Café (447 Poplar St.). The alley is named for the fourth bishop of Philadelphia and nicknamed Rosary Row because so many boys who lived here became priests.

At Lawrence Street, turn left. Continue to West Girard Avenue. The **9 National Shrine of St. John Neumann** displays the lifelike remains of the saint, who is credited with expanding the country's Catholic school system.

Turn left on West Girard Avenue. The mural on Haussemann's Pharmacy (536 W. Girard Ave.) honors the apothecary craft.

At North Seventh Street, turn left. The minister who founded Mt. Tabor African Methodist Episcopal Church (961–71 N. Seventh St.) in 1931 helped hardworking domestic workers who were being exploited by homeowners.

At Poplar Street, turn right. At Franklin Street, turn left. The Byzantine **10 Ukrainian Catholic Cathedral** was built in 1966 to resemble Istanbul's Hagia Sophia. A stone from Saint Peter the Apostle's tomb is part of the building, a gift from Pope Paul VI to symbolize unity between the two churches.

Continue to Brown Street and turn left. At North Seventh Street, turn right. The **11 Edgar Allan Poe National Historic Site** is where the author wrote "The Black Cat." Poe lived here with his wife and mother-in-law in 1843.

At Spring Garden Street, turn right to see Robert Venturi's **12 Guild House**, considered one of the most important works of the 20th century. Seriously. In *Twentieth-Century*

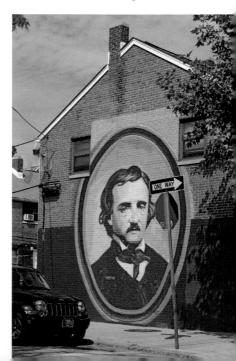

This mural of Edgar Allan Poe is near the home where Poe lived while writing "The Black Cat."

American Architecture: The Buildings and Their Makers, Carter Wiseman writes that the building combines historic forms with "banal" 20th-century commercialism, hiding a "slyly intellectual agenda" behind its "apparent ordinariness."

Turn around and walk east on Spring Garden Street. The ⑬ **German Society of Pennsylvania**, founded in 1764, has about 700 members. *Building America: German-American Contributions* (605 Spring Garden St.) acknowledges the German community's commitment.

Continue past 603 Spring Garden Street, where a ghost sign advertises LEATHER BELTING (for engines, not waists). Architect Frank Furness designed the former Northern Savings Fund Society Building (600 Spring Garden St.) in 1872.

⑭ The **Silk City Diner, Lounge and Garden,** is so named because the original stainless steel dining car placed here in 1954 was made in Paterson, New Jersey, then known as the Silk City.

The Value of Family on Northeast Treatment Centers (499 N. Fifth St.) highlights the center's work and features this George Bernard Shaw quote: "Perhaps the greatest social service that can be rendered by anybody to their country and to mankind is to bring up a family."

⑮ **Yards Brewing Company** has been making beer since 1994 and has taken inspiration from the Founding Fathers with "Ales of the Revolution." (The original brews had twice the alcohol content of today, as drinkers believed it better preserved the beer.) Varieties include Washington's Porter, which uses molasses to create a Philadelphia-style porter, and Poor Richard's Spruce Ale, based on a Benjamin Franklin recipe with barley, molasses, and spruce. Thomas Jefferson, who brewed beer at Monticello, once said beer could not be made by following a recipe, but the brewery still honored him with an ale with honey, wheat, and rye.

At North Fourth Street, turn left. Built in 1902, ⑯ **Integrity Trust Bank** was founded by three German immigrants and was one of the city's largest banking companies between 1880 and 1940, thanks to the many German brewers who entrusted their money to fellow community members.

The walk ends here. The River Wards tour (page 121) starts a few blocks from here at the Delaware River.

Points of Interest

① *Pedal Thru (Bikin' in the O-Zone)* 200 Spring Garden St.

② **Doughboy Park** N. Second and Spring Garden Sts.

③ **Standard Tap** 901 N. Second St., 215-238-0630, standardtap.com

(continued on next page)

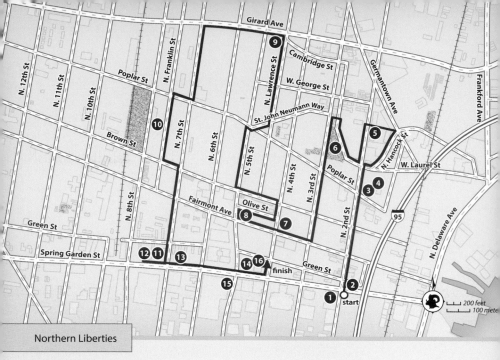

(continued from previous page)

④ **North Bowl** 909 N. Second St., 215-238-2695, northbowlphilly.com

⑤ **The Piazza** 1001 N. Second St., 215-987-5986, livepiazza.com

⑥ **Liberty Lands Park** 913 N. Third St., 215-627-6562, nlna.org/liberty-lands

⑦ **Saint Michael the Archangel Orthodox Church** 335 Fairmount Ave., 215-627-6148, saintmichaelsroc.org

⑧ **Saint Andrew's Russian Orthodox Cathedral** N. Fifth St. and Fairmount Ave., 215-627-3338, saintandrewscathedral.org

⑨ **The National Shrine of St. John Neumann** 1019 N. Fifth St., 215-627-3080, stjohnneumann.org

⑩ **Ukrainian Catholic Cathedral** 830 N. Franklin St., 215-922-2845, ukrcathedral.com

⑪ **Edgar Allan Poe National Historic Site** 532 N. Seventh St., 215-965-2305, nps.gov/edal

⑫ **Guild House** 711 Spring Garden St.

⑬ **German Society of Pennsylvania** 611 Spring Garden St.

⑭ **Silk City Diner, Lounge and Garden** 435 Spring Garden St., 215-592-8838, silkcityphilly.com

⑮ **Yards Brewing Company** 500 Spring Garden St., 215-525-0175, yardsbrewing.com

⑯ **Integrity Trust Bank** 542 N. Fourth St.

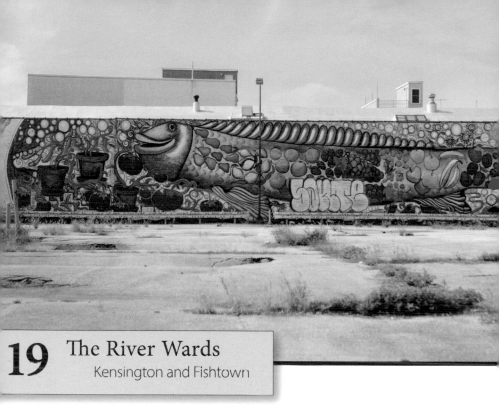

19 The River Wards
Kensington and Fishtown

Above: This Fishtown mural has become a neighborhood favorite.

BOUNDARIES: Delaware River, E. York St., Frankford Ave., Palmer Ave.
DISTANCE: 3.1 miles
DIFFICULTY: Easy
PARKING: Street parking is almost always available on side streets.
PUBLIC TRANSIT: SEPTA bus routes that stop nearby are 5, 25, 43, and MFL.

For years, outsiders considered Kensington dangerous, dirty, and plagued by problems. That would have shocked Anthony Palmer, who founded this once-independent city in the 1700s and named it after Kensington Palace. Many of the original street names referenced royalty. Girard Avenue, for example, was previously Prince Street.

In the 1800s, Kensington was safe and solid, home to blue-collar dock and factory workers. The decline began when the factories closed and picked up speed as the years passed.

The neighborhood's rebirth began in the late 20th century as artists and young people moved here, attracted by the low prices and the potential. Today transplants live side by side with families who have lived here for generations. Because of the creativity influx, walking these streets is a delight, with random art on walls, sidewalks, and even telephone poles. Fishtown is a small area within Kensington.

Walk Description

Begin at ❶ **Rivers Casino**. The gambling hall opened in 2010 after years of neighborhood protest. It was originally called Sugar House, a reference to the factory that once stood here. Construction uncovered remnants from a British fort and native relics dating back 3,000 years.

Facing the casino, turn left. At the intersection of North Delaware and Sugarhouse Drive, a ghost sign remembers the former Edward Corner Marine Merchandise Company.

Continue to Columbia Avenue. In the 1680s, William Penn signed a peace agreement with the native Lenni Lenape here at ❷ **Penn Treaty Park.** The deal was made in the shade of the Treaty Elm, which became a symbol of peace and love. The treaty was broken in 1755, when members of the Delaware tribe killed 24 settlers living nearby. Philadelphia leaders took revenge on the tribe for the next 300 years. The 7-acre park features picnic areas, a playground, and views of the Benjamin Franklin Bridge. A small museum is open by appointment.

Continue to the former ❸ **Delaware Power Station,** designed in the early 1900s by the architecture firm behind The Franklin Institute. It closed in 2004. It sits on historic land: the US Navy's first submarine—nicknamed Alligator because it was green—was built here in the 1860s. It moved via hand-cranked propeller. In 1863, the sub sunk during a violent storm while en route to provide underwater protection for Fort Sumter. It remains lost.

Backtrack to Columbia Avenue and turn right. At the North Delaware Street corner, *Under the Great Elm Shackamaxon* honors the treaty between Penn and the Lenni Lenape. Shackamaxon, which means "place of the council" was this area's native name.

At Allen Street, turn left. At Marlborough Street, turn right. Old Brick Church, also known as Kensington Methodist Church (300 Richmond St.), was in use from 1854 until it was sold in 2018 to a developer planning apartments. At its peak, the church welcomed more than 400 worshipers weekly. The current 20-member congregation has moved to a smaller building on the property.

Continue on Marlborough Street. At Girard Avenue, turn left. The Kensington Soup Society served meals to the hungry in a building nearby from 1844 to 2012. "Kensington Soup House" remains carved on the facade. During the winter of 1876–77, the organization fed about 28,000 people—an average of nearly 400 daily —according to the Preservation Alliance of Philadelphia. Those served included "families widowed or crippled by war, accident or disease; the unemployed; and workers whose wages could not cover the expenses of providing for their families. 'Bummers,' single men without fixed residence, were actively denied aid, as they were those suspected of 'double-dipping' from soup kitchens elsewhere in the city."

Pause at the corner of Girard and Frankford Avenues. The mural on the side of Garage North (100 E. Frankford Ave.) depicts Philadelphia 76ers shooting guard Matisse Thybulle. "BULL" is highlighted, as this is an ad for a popular energy drink. Look across Frankford Avenue. The Wells Fargo bank (1148 Frankford Ave.) opened in 1878 as the Kensington National Bank and was designed by noted architect Frank Furness. A 2021 redevelopment proposal for the block would renovate the interior and exterior and add residential and retail space.

Turn right on Frankford, crossing Girard Avenue to ❹ **Johnny Brenda's.** In the 1960s, a boxer named Johnny Imbrenda ran a rough neighborhood bar here. In the early 2000s, two experienced restaurateurs purchased the place despite the questionable neighborhood and rebranded the spot as a music venue with gastropub leanings. It reopened in 2003 and helped launch the neighborhood's renaissance.

Continue on Frankford Avenue. The mural on ❺ **Cake Life Bake Shop,** *We Are Universal,* celebrates transgender and nonbinary Philadelphians and was designed with input from youth living at Morris Homes, the nation's only recovery program for trans and gender-nonconforming individuals. It includes their answers to the questions, "What do you want people to get out of this mural? What is really important about the culture of Morris Homes that you want people to know?"

Across the street is ❻ **Fishtown Tavern**. Fishtown is part of Kensington, so named because of the many commercial fishermen who lived here, working the shad-filled Delaware River, writes Kenneth Milano in *Remembering Kensington and Fishtown: The Story of a Philadelphia River Ward.* Look for fish imagery in sidewalk imprints, in ironwork, on telephone poles, and on residential house number plates. Many trashcans have an opening shaped like a fish's mouth. The neighborhood's original residents were known for their pride of place, and the newest residents share that.

Continue walking. ❼ **La Colombe** is arguably the best coffee in the city.

❽ **Lutheran Settlement House,** founded in 1902, continues to serve vulnerable men, women, and children with a variety of services. Two murals of note here: Outside, *Settlement House Roots,* which features glass mosaic flowers popping off the wall, honors employees and the people they serve. Inside is *You Are Not Alone*, which looks like a stained glass window. The words "I am not what happened to me" are above a portrait of Mark Hudson, who was shot and killed in 2015. Mark's mother, Karen, works with Settlement House. Her voice trembled with emotion when the mural was completed. "Mark is still bigger than life and I'm just overjoyed to see him living forever," she said.

The garden next to Settlement House is part of Wm. Mulherin's Sons, 1355 E. Front St., a restaurant and bar housed in a converted whiskey factory. The Mulherins made whiskey here from 1900 to 1924, shipping it via horse and wagon.

To create *Persistence* (1412 Frankford Ave.), Jason Andrew Turner partnered with women from Lutheran Settlement House. The project's manager told streetsdept.com that "The portrait does not portray an existing person in the present, but rather one deeply inspired by the oral history of long-time community members and the history of LSH."

The building that now houses Cheu Noodle Bar (1416 Frankford Ave.) was constructed in 1892 for the 10th District Patrol House, an example of "the Police Bureau's commitment to enlarging its services citywide with construction of police stations and patrol houses," according to the Philadelphia Register of Historic Places. It was used until 1950.

The pocket park at 1405 Frankford Avenue at Belgrade Street is a memorial to resident Wayne Elliss Jr., who was shot and killed nearby in 2002. A 2020 transformation added benches, pavers, and plants.

Continue on Frankford Avenue. **9 Heffe**, a walk-up taco shop, replaced a gas station. Try the fried octopus tacos with tomato jam. The brightly painted Peace A Pie (1429 Marlborough St.) is a regional chain that invites visitors to "Live. Love. Local."

At Frankford Avenue and Palmer Street, Palmer Park is named after Kensington's founder. The Fishtown Neighbors Association keeps this tiny park hopping with events, including movie nights and a farmers market.

10 *You Can Be Stronger Than Diabetes* covers the Bell Surplus Floor Covering warehouse. Drug manufacturing company GlaxoSmithKline sponsored the mural as part of a public education project after statistics showed this neighborhood had the city's highest rate of diabetes diagnoses in people ages 18 and younger. The mural promotes healthy eating, with images of fruits and vegetables inside a fish-shaped outline.

Neumann Medical Center (1601 E. Palmer St.) was once the 80-bed St. Mary's Hospital, run by the Order of the Sisters of St. Francis. (Take a look down Palmer Street to see the original name carved above an entrance.) In the 1840s, the Philadelphia archdiocese sent three nuns here to help the poor and infirm. The need was so great that in five years the nuns treated more than 15,000 patients, mostly German and Irish immigrants. The hospital's constitution was written in German.

The park at 1825 Frankford Avenue was a trash-filled lot until leaders of the New Kensington CDC and residents spent six weeks reclaiming the property in 1997. It can be rented as event space.

Made and Maker (2021 Frankford Ave.) is a women-owned store selling vintage items and works by local artists and makers. It was featured on Netflix's makeover show *Queer Eye* in 2020.

Continuing on Frankford Avenue, **⑪ Pizza Brain** offers pizza by the pie or the slice. The restaurant is also the home of the Museum of Pizza Culture, which has the world's largest collection of pizza-related memorabilia, as certified by the Guinness World Records.

At East York Street, turn right. Horatio B. Hackett Elementary School (2161 E. York St.) is named for an American biblical scholar who died in 1875. Note its front mosaic and the ABC mural wrapping around the side and rear of the building.

The corner property at 2176 E. York Street is another work by Frank Furness. It was completed in 1886 for "John Ruhl, a conveyer and Councilman turned criminal" who stole at least $30,000 from his employers, its Philadelphia Register of Historic Places application notes. The form speculates that Ruhl took money to pay his gambling debts, quoting a newspaper article that asserts Ruhl "was a heavy poker player at the Vesta Club and a big loser." Ruhl did time at Eastern State Penitentiary. In 2022, the nearly 5,000-square-foot home was valued at $1.3 million.

At Sepviva Street, turn right. Konrad Square Park is named for firefighter Joseph Konrad, who was killed on the job in 1984.

At East Dauphin Street, turn left, passing Summerfield-Siloam United Methodist Church (2223 E. Dauphin St.), which was built in 1911.

Continue on East Dauphin Street. The next two blocks look unlike any others on this walk, with set-back homes, lots of greenery, and a mix of old and new construction.

At Cedar Street, turn right. At E. Berks St., turn right again. St. Laurentius Roman Catholic Church, which stood here, was funded by Polish immigrants who contributed every spare nickel and dime to build it in 1885. It was scheduled for demolition in summer 2022.

Turn left on Memphis Street and continue to **⑫ Palmer Cemetery**. Neighborhood founder Palmer established this 5-acre cemetery as a free final resting place for locals. (Cremains preferred.) It's still active, offering free space to current residents or property owners. A monument inside remembers Mary Ann and John Willingmyre's five sons who fought in the Civil War, according to palmercemeteryfishtown.com. Two were killed, two were wounded, and one was captured. Palmer himself lies in Christ Church Cemetery with Ben Franklin.

At East Palmer Street, turn left. At Girard Avenue, turn right. **⑬ First Presbyterian Church,** another neighborhood landmark, was built in 1859. The structure originally had a 180-foot-tall steeple, but it deteriorated and was replaced with the copper dome in the 1920s.

This walk ends here, near where it began. The start of the Northern Liberties tour (page 114) is 1 mile away.

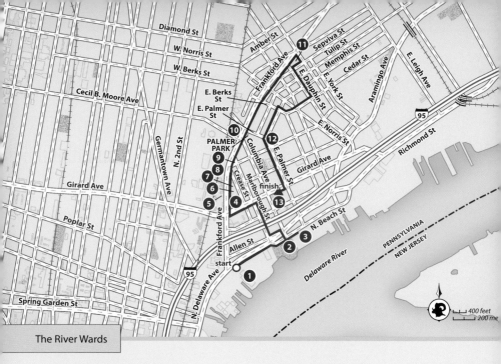

Points of Interest

- **1**   **Rivers Casino**   1001 N. Delaware Ave., 877-477-3715, riverscasino.com
- **2**   **Penn Treaty Park**   1199 N. Delaware Ave., delawareriverwaterfront.com
- **3**   **Delaware Power Station**   1325 Beach St.
- **4**   **Johnny Brenda's**   1201 Frankford Ave., 215-739-9684, johnnybrendas.com
- **5**   **Cake Life Bake Shop**   1306 Frankford Ave., 215-268-7343, cakelifebakeshop.com
- **6**   **Fishtown Tavern**   1301 Frankford Ave., 267-687-8406, fishtowntavern.com
- **7**   **La Colombe**   1335 Frankford Ave., 267-479-1600, lacolombe.com
- **8**   **Lutheran Settlement House**   1340 Frankford Ave., 215-426-8610, lutheransettlement.org
- **9**   **Heffe**   1431 Frankford Ave., 215-423-2309, heffetacos.com
- **10**   *You Can Be Stronger Than Diabetes*   1706 Frankford Ave.
- **11**   **Pizza Brain**   2313 Frankford Ave., 215-291-2965, pizzabrain.org
- **12**   **Palmer Cemetery**   1499 E. Palmer St.
- **13**   **First Presbyterian Church**   410–22 E.Girard Ave.

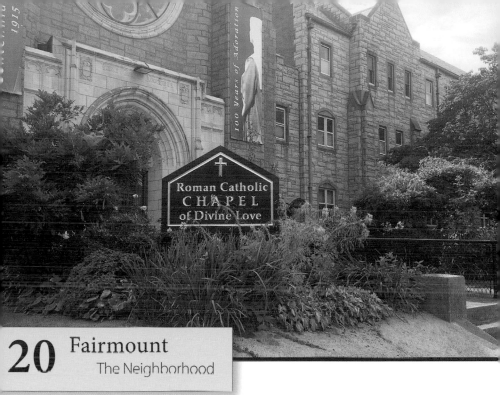

20 Fairmount
The Neighborhood

Above: The Holy Spirit Adoration sisters are cloistered nuns known as the pink sisters because of their rose-colored habits.

BOUNDARIES: W. Girard Ave., Spring Garden St., N. Broad St., N. 25th St.
DISTANCE: 3.7 miles
DIFFICULTY: Easy, with downhill stretches
PARKING: Street parking is usually available unless a special event is taking place; there's a paid lot at N. 22nd St. and Fairmount Ave.
PUBLIC TRANSIT: SEPTA's Broad Street subway line takes you to Fairmount's eastern border. Bus lines include the 7, 32, 33, and 48.

William Penn named this neighborhood northwest of Center City for the high hill, or "fair mount" on which it sits, giving residents a great view of the Schuylkill River. It's called the Art Museum area by many because of its proximity to that landmark. The area closer to downtown is also known as Spring Garden.

Walk Description

Begin at Greater Exodus Baptist Church (704 N. Broad St.), built in 1877. Its minister, former Philadelphia Eagle Herbert H. Lusk II, was given the nickname "The Praying Tailback" in college because he would go down on one knee, lower his head, and pray. As he told philadelphiaeagles.com, it was his way of thanking God for helping him heal from a junior college knee injury. "Doctors said I'd never play football again, but I put my faith in God's hands . . . I knew if my knee healed, it was His will for me to continue playing." Lusk became the minister here in 1982 and now leads a 2,000-member-strong congregation.

Facing the church, turn left. The building at the corner of North Broad Street and Ridge Avenue was constructed in 1918 for the Northwestern National Bank. In 1949, it became the first city bank to have a drive-through teller window. It changed hands multiple times, with each owner putting panels with the bank's new name over the old name. Greater Exodus Baptist Church purchased the deteriorating building for $1 and reopened it as the nonprofit People for People Inc., which offers a community credit union.

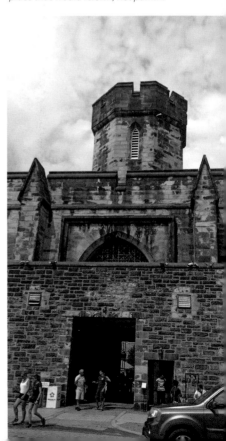

Eastern State Penitentiary was conceived as a place that would reform, not punish.

Cross Ridge Avenue and turn left to reach ❶ **JBJ Soul Homes** at Fairmount and Ridge Avenues. Local nonprofit Project Home partnered with rocker Jon Bon Jovi to build this four-story, mixed-use building with 55 apartments for formerly homeless and low-income people. Artist Meg Saligman created the two-story mural *Fire Beacon,* which contains a round glass sculpture that is lit at night. Inside, one lobby wall contains a line from a song on Bon Jovi's ninth album, "Who says you can't go home?"

Leave North Broad Street behind and walk west on Fairmount Avenue. Overseas Motor Works (1501–05 Fairmount Ave.) is a 1930s Art

Deco building specifically designed to house an auto-related business when North Broad Street was known as automobile row.

Project Home resident Vanise Clay designed *The Watchers* on the side of 1515 Fairmount Avenue. Artist Robert Bullock did the actual painting.

HOMEspun Boutique (1523 Fairmount Ave.) sells used clothing and products made by Project Home residents, including soap and candles. It's staffed by people who have experienced homelessness.

Cross North 16th Street. The murals on Jobbers Warehouse (1601 Fairmount Ave.) encourage voting in the 2020 presidential election. The top floor panel above the door shows a Quaker or Colonial figure holding a tire.

Continue on Fairmount Avenue. Built in 1901, the A. F. Bornot Brothers Dye Works Building (1642 Fairmount Ave.) opened as a mixed-use residential and retail building in 2016.

Cross North 17th Street. In 2021, a demolition permit was issued for the warehouse/beer distributor at 1701 Fairmount Avenue, which phillyyimby.com called "a welcome streetscape improvement."

Continue to Corinthian Avenue. ❷ **Eastern State Penitentiary** opened in 1829 and was conceived as a true penitentiary, one that would reform, not punish. The cells were lit by skylights in the vaulted ceilings, the message being that only God and hard work could provide redemption.

Among the big-name criminals held here were bank robber Willie Sutton and gangster Al Capone. The penitentiary closed in 1970. The nonprofit that runs the site examines the development of the criminal justice system. One exhibition showed how incarceration has negatively affected the nation. The site offers tours and hosts an annual Halloween haunted house to finance its programming.

Turn right on Corinthian Avenue. The greenery on the penitentiary's east side is the Corinthian Gardens, opened to the public in 2020. For years, this space was bare and trash-filled. Neighbors formed Friends of Eastern State Penitentiary in 1996 and created this space, which includes community garden plots and recreation spaces.

Continue on Corinthian Avenue. The Grand Corinthian (909 Corinthian Ave.) was built in 1911 and for decades was a dormitory for nurses working nearby. It was converted to apartments in the second half of the 20th century and was completely renovated in 2021.

The white building ahead is ❸ **Girard College's Founder's Hall**, considered one of the country's finest examples of Greek Revival architecture. Banker/merchant Stephen Girard was one of the richest men in the country when he died in 1831. His fortune established Girard College, a school for poor, white, male orphans, many of whom were the sons of coal miners, which opened in 1833.

Today the school is open to both genders and all skin hues and offers full scholarships and boarding for academically gifted students from families of limited means.

Turn right on Girard Avenue. The Smith Chapel Baptist Church (1828 Ridge Ave.) was built in the 1880s as Northwestern National Bank. Philaphilia.blogspot.com says the building's architect is unknown but notes, "This little building kicks ass. It can't be easy to pull off a good design on a triangular shaped lot. You got to love the massive entranceway, like you're going to enter Valhalla every time you go to the bank." The church has occupied the building since 1969.

Turn left on Ridge Avenue. ④ **St. Joseph's Preparatory School** is a private Jesuit school that had 95 students when it opened in 1851. In 1966, a fire razed two-thirds of the school. When it reopened a few years later, the school's website says, "the marble stairs from the old building had been buried under the glass and slate foyer to signify the strength of the Prep."

At North College Avenue, turn left. ⑤ *Henry Ossawa Tanner: Letters of Influence* honors a man described as "the Jackie Robinson of the art world, the Barack Obama of painting." Tanner, who died in 1937, was one of the first African American artists to receive international acclaim. The mural was created with adjudicated male youths living in detention.

Stephen Girard is at the center of this sculpture on the grounds of the school he founded.

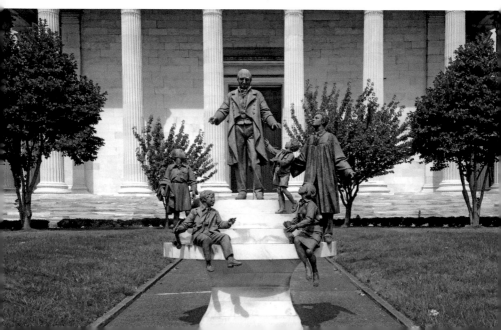

Continue on North College Avenue, passing *Cancer Support for Life* (N. College Ave. and 22nd St.), which features cancer survivors and the people who support them.

The historical marker for the Dixie Hummingbirds (25th St. near N. College Ave.) sits outside the former home of James Davis, who founded the band in 1929. The Birds, as they were often called, were an influential gospel group, with artists including James Brown, Paul Simon, and Jackie Wilson citing the band as an influence. When the marker was placed in 2017, the oldest surviving Dixie Hummingbird, Howard Carroll, 93, told *The Philadelphia Tribune* he was happy the band was to be honored, saying Davis "made sure we always carried ourselves as gentlemen. That's why we were called the gentlemen of song." The Birds won the 1973 Best Soul Gospel Performance for "Loves Me Like A Rock."

Moving Forward, 2521 W. College Ave., looks at the neighborhood's history and the changing community, featuring images of current residents, local architecture, and the Route 15 Trolley.

At West College Avenue, turn left. At Poplar Street, turn left again, passing St. Nicholas Ukrainian Catholic Church (871 N. 24th St.). After World War II, eastern Europeans built a wooden church here in the 1950s. This brick structure rose in 1978.

At North 24th Street, turn right. At Aspen Street, turn right. Patrick Ward Memorial Park (24th and Aspen Sts.) is named for a 21-year-old neighborhood resident killed in the Vietnam War while serving as a helicopter gunner. A 1997 *Philadelphia Inquirer* article described neighbors watching the brown Army car slowly move down the narrow street to the Ward home.

Continue on Aspen Street. The ❻ **former home of director David Lynch** was the location for *The Alphabet,* his first 4 minute film. Some people call this area "Eraserhood," a reference to Lynch's 1977 film *Eraserhead.* A 2015 BillyPenn.com article notes that this is where Lynch got his inspiration for the "dark, surrealist horror film about a man who lives alone in an apartment in a post-industrial area." Lynch also said that "Philadelphia—this area specifically—scared the hell out of him."

The house was built as a Trinity, also called a Father, Son, Holy Ghost house. These homes typically have three floors with one room on each floor connected by winding staircases and a basement kitchen. Most are smaller than 1,000 square feet. Servants and lower-income workers typically lived in these homes.

At North 25th Street, turn left, passing Philly Fairmount Art Center (2501 Olive St.), a neighborhood hub. At Fairmount Avenue, turn left.

At North 23rd Street, turn right. Walk to Wallace Street and turn right again. At North 24th Street, turn left, walking down Penn's "fair mount." At Green Street, turn left. ❼ **St. Francis Xavier Church** was founded in 1839. The Philadelphia Congregation of the Oratory, a group of secular priests who have served the community since 1990, are based here.

Continue on Green Street. Prepare for serious house envy. The Romanesque brownstone at 2220 Green Street belongs to former Pennsylvania state senator Vincent J. Fumo, who in 2009 was convicted of more than 135 federal corruption charges. Built in the 1880s, the 33-room, 19,200-square-foot mansion has six bedrooms and 10 bathrooms, a wine cellar, a shooting range, and servants' quarters.

Fumo was in a federal prison until August 2013, then served the rest of his time at home. One newspaper reporter called this building "the federal correctional institution at Fairmount, also known as the Fumo mansion."

The **❽ Bergdoll Mansion** has eight bedrooms, nine bathrooms, two kitchens, and hand-painted ceilings. During World War I, Grover Cleveland Bergdoll, grandson of the original owner, lived here with his mother. According to philly.curbed.com, when World War I began, Bergdoll "dodged the draft . . . by hiding in the mansion."

Bergdoll escaped to Germany, living well on his family's fortune. When he was found by bounty hunters, he killed one and bit the thumb off the other, earning the nickname the Fighting Slacker. In May 1939, Bergdoll returned to the United States—but only to avoid being drafted into the Nazi Army.

Continue on Green Street. The Chapel of Divine Love and the convent of the **❾ Holy Spirit Adoration Sisters** is home to cloistered nuns called the pink sisters because they wear rose-colored habits to signify the joy they feel honoring the Holy Spirit. The chapel never closes, and at least one nun has been in prayer nonstop since 1915.

Continue on Green Street, stopping at North 20th Street. In the 1970s, the Reverend Gabriel Real, pastor of Our Lady of the Miraculous Medal Church, spearheaded the building of these eight yellow structures for low-income congregants. The homes in Spanish Village cost $20,000, but a family could make a down payment as low as $200.

At North 19th Street, turn left. St. Andrew Lithuanian Catholic Church (1911 Wallace St.) offers services in Lithuanian and English.

Cross North 19th Street. Sculptor Evelyn Keyser's *People Pyramid*, installed in 1971, shows "members of a family supporting one another, with fathers on the bottom tier, sons on the second tier and their brothers on the top," website creativephl.org notes.

Spring Gardens at Wallace Street provides space to almost 200 local families and serves as an outdoor classroom, hosting cooking and planting workshops.

❿ Roberto Clemente Park was the heart of the neighborhood's Puerto Rican community, which reached its population peak in the 1970s. Locals fell asleep to the sounds of Puerto Rican music performed here by the 20Gs, a local gang that served as the neighborhood's protectors. As this area changed and property values increased, many of these residents moved, returning for the annual Clemente Fest.

Continue east on Wallace Street. *Tribute to Diego Rivera* (N. 17th and Wallace Sts.) is divided into three sections, each representing a different theme prominent in Rivera's art: the working man, the community, and the family.

At North 17th Street, turn right. At Mt. Vernon Street, turn right again. The former church at 1722 Mt. Vernon Street is a condominium building called The Church. The ⓫ home of Thomas Eakins is now the headquarters of Mural Arts Philadelphia, the city-affiliated nonprofit responsible for most city murals. Eakins was a realist painter, photographer, and sculptor, and one of the most important modern American artists. The green space in front of the Philadelphia Museum of Art is named for him.

Continue to North 18th Street and turn left. Laura W. Waring School is named for the well-known African American artist whose 1944 exhibition *Portraits of Outstanding Citizens of Negro Origin* included a painting of Marian Anderson. Many Waring paintings are in the National Portrait Gallery's permanent collection. The floral mosaic flanking the school's side doors is *Doorway to Imagination*.

Continue to Spring Garden Street. ⓬ Highway Tabernacle began as a gospel wagon in 1895, with local preachers traveling from town to town. After four months, they had stopped 35 times and spoken to about 35,000 people. The next year they were even busier. They established the original church soon after. After a 1986 fire destroyed the building, congregants gathered to sing and pray. When a reporter asked how people could be so happy looking at the burnt building, one woman replied, "We don't cry over things; we cry over people."

Turn left. The ⓭ former Stetson Mansion, now condos, was the home of hat magnate John B. Stetson, whose famous hats were manufactured in Philadelphia.

The New Jersey–born son of a hatmaker, Stetson traveled through the American West before settling here in 1865. His travels and observations led to his hat's unique design. The *Dictionary of the American West* includes this description from a Stetson fan: "It kept the sun out of your eyes and off your neck. It was an umbrella. It gave you a bucket (the crown) to water your horse and a cup (the brim) to water yourself. It made a hell of a fan, which you need sometimes for a fire but more often to shunt cows this direction or that."

This walk ends here. North Broad Street is just three blocks away. See pages 45 and 53 for those tours.

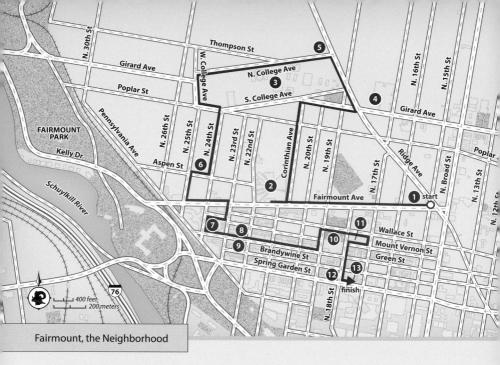

Fairmount, the Neighborhood

Points of Interest

1 **Project Home/JBJ Soul Homes** 1415 Fairmount Ave. and 1515 Fairmount Ave., 215-232-7272, projecthome.org

2 **Eastern State Penitentiary** 2027 Fairmount Ave, 215-236-3300, easternstate.org

3 **Girard College** 2101 S. College Ave., 215-787-2600, girardcollege.edu

4 **St. Joseph's Preparatory School** 1733 W. Girard Ave., 215-978-1950, sjprep.org

5 *Henry Ossawa Tanner: Letters of Influence* 2019 N. College Ave. Mural Arts Philadelphia, 215-685-0750, muralarts.org.

6 **Former home of director David Lynch** 2429 Aspen St.

7 **St. Francis Xavier Church** 2319 Green St., 215-765-4568, sfxoratory.org

8 **Bergdoll Mansion** 2201 Green St.

9 **Holy Spirit Adoration Sisters** 2212 Green St., 215-567-0123, adorationsisters.org

10 **Roberto Clemente Park** N. 19th and Wallace Sts., myphillypark.org/explore/parks /clemente-park-playground

11 **Former home of Thomas Eakins** 1729 Mt. Vernon St. Mural Arts Philadelphia, 215-685-0750, muralarts.org.

12 **Highway Tabernacle** 1801 Spring Garden St., 215-563-9192, highwaytabernacle.org

13 **Former Stetson Mansion** 1717 Spring Garden St.

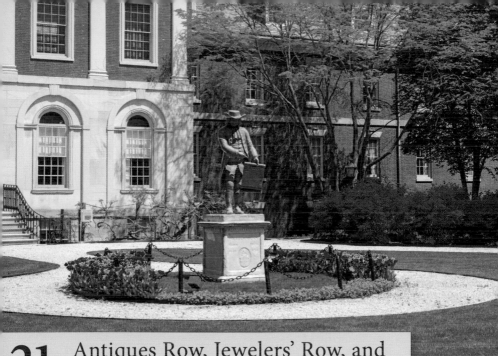

21 Antiques Row, Jewelers' Row, and Rittenhouse Row
A Cross Section of the City in Less Than 3 Miles

BOUNDARIES: Schuylkill River, S. Sixth St., Pine St., Chestnut St.
DISTANCE: 2.7 miles
DIFFICULTY: Easy
PARKING: There are multiple pay lots throughout this walk, as well as street parking.
PUBLIC TRANSIT: Crosstown buses run back and forth on Pine St., where this tour begins, and Lombard St., one block south of Pine. Consider the 12, 40, and 42.

This Center City walk includes the nation's first hospital, oldest diamond district, and two of the city's most upscale clothing stores.

Walk Description

Start at ❶ **Louis I. Kahn Park.** When Kahn died in 1974 at age 73, he was the country's most celebrated architect, as a *New Yorker* piece later noted. The park, established in the 1970s, was originally "a low maintenance space with few plantings, earning it the nickname, 'Concrete Park,'" notes the Friends of Louis I. Kahn group, which has created a much more welcome space.

Head east on Pine Street. The stretch between 9th and 11th Streets has been called "Antiques Row" for decades. Amy Finkel, whose family store is the next stop on this walk, told hiddencity phila.org in 2012 that when her father opened his shop in 1947, "There was no question. If you wanted to open an antiques business, this was the place to be then." Today, only a handful of antiques businesses remain.

Head east on Pine Street. ❷ **M. Finkel & Daughter** specializes in 18th- and 19th-century needlework. Current owner Amy Finkel told hiddencityphila.org in 2012 that when her father opened his shop in 1947, "There was no question. If you wanted to open an antiques business, this was the place to be then." Today, only a handful of antiques businesses remain. Antiquing is different in the Internet age: After acquiring a sampler made in 1832 by an 8-year-old English girl named Thisbe Danson, Finkel easily found Thisbe's descendant in England. The man purchased the sampler and now owns something created by his ancestor via a Philadelphia shopkeeper.

Continue east to the nation's first hospital, ❸ **Pennsylvania Hospital.** Other firsts here include the first general vaccine against pneumonia, the first use of intravenous feeding, and the development of magnetic resonance imaging (MRI). Dr. Thomas Bond and Benjamin Franklin founded the hospital in 1751. It's open for guided and self-guided tours.

A statue of city founder William Penn stands at the center of the Physic Garden, Eighth and Pine Streets. Rumor is his ghost leaves the statue and walks the grounds at night.

Turn left on South Eighth Street. At Delancey Street, pass the 1938 Richard H. Harte Memorial Building. Harte earned the army's Distinguished Service Medal during World War I for being "one of the pioneering instructors in the principles of battle surgery."

Continue on South Eighth Street. At Locust Street, turn right. Ahead is ❹ **Washington Square,** one of the city's original green spaces. The square holds the Tomb of the Unknown Revolutionary War Soldier, and many soldiers are buried under this square.

Continue to the corner. The Farm Journal Building (230 W. Washington Square) has a stone cornucopia above its entrance. In print since 1827, the publication, now published elsewhere, remains the country's largest farming magazine.

Follow the square to the corner of St. James Street to find The Ayer, a condo building that once housed the advertising firm of N. W. Ayer & Son. Founded in 1869, the company's memorable slogans include "A Diamond is Forever" and "Be All that You Can Be."

Bear right, following the park. At Walnut Street, turn right. **5 The Curtis Building** housed the Curtis Publishing Company, one of the country's largest publishers in the early 1900s. It printed *Ladies' Home Journal, Jack and Jill,* and *The Saturday Evening Post.* The interior features a waterfall and Maxwell Parrish's mosaic *Dream Garden,* which contains more than 100,000 pieces of glass and is seen in *The Sixth Sense.*

At Sixth Street, turn left. **6 The Public Ledger Building** housed the daily newspaper that was known for its bold, tabloid-style headlines and rhyming obituaries. The penny paper, launched in 1836, almost folded when management opposed the Civil War. New owners rebranded it as a Union supporter and it once again flourished. Its presses—the country's first rotary ones, which quadrupled the printing speed—shut down in 1942. The site of publisher George W. Childs's mansion, now demolished, appears later in this walk.

At Chestnut Street, turn left. The sidewalk features plaques commemorating the 56 signers of the Declaration of Independence. Continue to South Seventh Street and turn left. Walk one block to Samson Street and turn right. Jewelers' Row, which runs from Walnut to Market Streets and South Seventh to South Ninth Streets, has about 300 retailers, wholesalers, and jewelry craftspeople. It's the country's oldest diamond district, dating to 1851.

Continue to South Eighth Street. The marker at the **7 Craftsman Row Saloon** honors Robert Bogle, an African American man who had a thriving catering business. A 1987 *Philadelphia Inquirer* article described Bogle as a favorite of wealthy Nicholas Biddle. "Of the two dozen or so catering dynasties that sprang up in the city in the 1800s . . . a disproportionate number were founded by blacks," the article said. "At a time when most blacks found little or no opportunity to advance, the black caterers achieved money, power—even in some cases, a measure of immortality." When Bogle died, Biddle penned an "Ode to Bogle," suggesting "no human ritual, be it marriage, christening, or even death, was complete if not attended to by the stern, multifarious Bogle."

Head south on South Eighth Street. At Walnut Street, turn right. **8 The Walnut Street Theatre,** founded in 1809, is the country's oldest English-speaking theater. The Marquis de Lafayette and President Thomas Jefferson were in the audience for its first production. The Walnut was the first theater to install gas footlights (1837) and the first to have air-conditioning (1855).

Across Walnut, **9 Wills Eye Hospital,** established in 1834, is the country's oldest continuously operating eye-care center. Quaker merchant James Wills Jr. donated $116,000 to found it.

Brower Hatcher's *Starman in the Ancient Garden* sculpture depicts a spaceship that has crash-landed. The artist wanted the work to provoke viewers to reflect on "what we have been, what we are, and what we may become."

Continue on Walnut Street, crossing South Tenth Street to the campus of Jefferson University Hospital and Medical School, founded in 1824 when only four colleges offered medical training. Alums include 1828 graduate Samuel D. Gross, one of the finest surgeons of his time.

Pass the first building to see sculptor Henry Weber Mitchell's *The Winged Ox* atop a pedestal engraved with names of famous healers. The fictional creature is a symbol of St. Luke the physician. To take a quick break, turn left at the statue and relax in the campus green space. The fountain depicting frolicking otters at the entrance is another Mitchell sculpture.

Continue west. Sculptor Jim Sanborn's cylindrical *Ars Medendi*—Latin for "Medical Arts"—features historic medical texts from around the world. When the statue's lit at night, the words are projected onto the surrounding sidewalk.

Cross South Eleventh Street. **10 The Forrest Theatre** is named for noted American thespian Edwin Forrest. Forrest's long feud with British actor William Macready caused New York's 1849 Astor Place Riot, which left 22 dead and 100 injured.

Short version: Forrest was the darling of the working class, while Macready's supporters were largely upper-class Anglophiles. In 1849, a group of Forrest's supporters attended Macready's performance of *Macbeth* at Astor Place Theater and shut down the performance by pummeling the stage with rotten eggs, potatoes, lemons, and shoes. When Macready performed again three days later, fights broke out among fans of both men outside the venue.

Continue west. The striking 26-story luxury apartment building at 1213 Walnut Street,

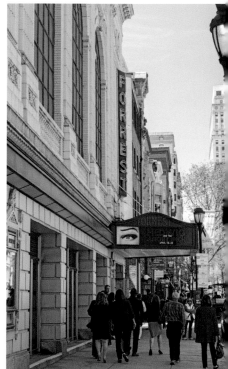

The Forrest Theatre is named for actor Edwin Forrest.

completed in 2017, offers amenities including a dog run and a community terrace. The two-story lobby features wood accents made of . . . walnut.

11 **The Witherspoon Building** fills the entire city block between Walnut, Sansom, S. Broad, and S. Juniper Streets. It exemplifies the "more is more" school of design. Built in 1897 as the Presbyterian Board of Publications and Sabbath School, the structure is covered with medallions and sculptures of historic figures. The National Register of Historic Places calls each of its entrances "a showcase of sculpture." (Make a right for a quick detour on Juniper Street to fully appreciate that assessment.) Architect James Huston wanted "to tell the story of the Organization of the Presbyterian Church in this country in Architecture, Painting, and Sculpture." It's named for John Witherspoon, the only Presbyterian minister to sign the Declaration of Independence.

Continue west on Walnut Street. The **12** **Bellevue-Stratford Hotel** was once one of the country's most glamorous hotels, hosting two Republican National Conventions, a Democratic National Convention, and an American Legion conference that ended with an outbreak of Legionnaire's disease.

Cross Broad Street. This stretch of Walnut Street was once called Bank Row. First Pennsylvania Bank, founded in 1782, occupied the corner building at 1401 Broad. The original home for the Philadelphia Stock Exchange was 1411. The Drexel building at 1435 was built in 1926 for bankers Drexel and Company.

Butcher and Singer steakhouse (1500 Walnut St.) replaced First National Bank, which in 1863 was the first commercial bank to print a federal bank note. (The bank's president then bought horses for the First Troop Philadelphia Cavalry so it could deploy to Gettysburg.) The Stock Brokerage House of Hano, Wasserman & Co. stood at 1513 Walnut, while Industrial Valley Bank greeted visitors to 1518 with a spread-winged gold eagle above the arched door.

The Art Deco **13** **Icon**, a retail/residential building, is marketed as "wellness real estate," meaning residences offer vitamin C-infused showers and lighting that regulates melatonin levels. When the structure was completed in 1929, it was considered an architectural marvel and its five-story parking garage was a novelty.

Three 19th-century properties in the 1700 block of Walnut Street were damaged in May of 2020 during the civic uprising after George Floyd's murder in Minneapolis. Originally built as private homes, the three properties were converted to retail in the early 1900s. The future of this space is in doubt.

Continue to South 18th Street. To the left is Rittenhouse Square. Across the street is the Beaux Arts mansion commissioned in 1898 by Sarah Drexel Fell, the widow of a coal magnate, for herself and her new husband, Alexander Van Renssalaer. The Anthropologie store retains its ornate staircase, stained glass dome, and a ceiling covered with paintings of Italian royalty in gold frames.

Turn right on South 18th Street. InnerVision Fine Eyewear (131 S. 18th St.) occupies the former home of construction magnate Allen Rorke, whose projects included Philadelphia's Bourse Building and the Pennsylvania State Capital. *The Philadelphia Times* called him "the nation's greatest builder." When Rorke died in 1899 at age 53, many estimated his estate at more than $1 million. Instead, his heirs collected $952.56.

Continue north. The private residence at 122 South 18th Street was built and designed by the influential firm of Cope and Stewardson, best known for Collegiate Gothic buildings on the campuses of Bryn Mawr College, Princeton University, and the University of Pennsylvania.

At Chestnut Street, turn left. The Belgravia (1811 Chestnut St.) was originally the Belgravia Hotel, opened in 1902. Efram Zimbalist, who at age 21 in 1909 was considered the world's greatest violinist, lived here, as did soprano Alma Gluck. The intricate façade of terra cotta, granite, and brick was restored in 2016.

⑭ Boyd's opened in 1938 as a custom shirt shop, replacing a funeral home. It sells custom suits, which can cost more than $5,000. The founder's grandchildren run the business and employ a team of more than 25 staff tailors.

At South 19th Street, turn left. Sophy Curson opened her eponymous clothing boutique at 122 S. 19th Street in 1929. Curson was less than 5 feet tall, and the store initially specialized in dressing petite women. Her patented logo was "Junior is a size, not an age." The third generation of her family now runs the business.

At Sansom Street, turn right. *Summer Rendezvous,* on the second floor of Shake Shack (2000 Sansom St.), brings some greenery to a concrete-heavy corner.

Continue west, passing the Roxy Theater (2023 Sansom) and the Adrienne Theater (2030 Sansom). At South 21st Street, turn left. Continue to Walnut Street. Ahead the **⑮ First Presbyterian Church** features Tiffany stained glass windows from 1872.

Turn right on Walnut Street. *The Public Ledger*'s publisher, George W. Childs, lived in an opulent mansion at 2128 Walnut Street. The home was torn down in 1970.

Cross South 22nd Street, noting how the wall overlooking the gas station has trompe l'oeil murals resembling church windows. The Art Deco residential building at 2212 Walnut Street was the headquarters of WPEN, AM 950. The station dominated the airwaves in the 1950s, with popular programs including *Mambo Dance Party* hosted by Al I Raymond aka "Pancho the Man in the Black Sombrero." In the 1960s, the station hosted an interview show with musicians

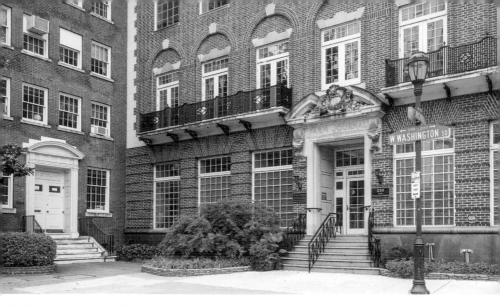

The Farm Journal *was published in this urban setting for more than 100 years.*

in its small first-floor restaurant, allowing people to walk in and see stars such as Frank Zappa and Jerry Lewis.

Continue on Walnut Street, crossing South 23rd Street and walking halfway across the Schuylkill River bridge. Turn around to see *The Phillies Mural* (24th and Walnut Sts.), which honors the 1980 and 2008 World Series champions.

Look left. In 2013, Freeman's Auctions (2400 Market St.) offered the original ransom notes sent to the parents of Charley Ross, a four-year-old taken from outside his parent's Germantown home in July 1874. He was the country's first kidnap victim.

In sloppily written letters filled with misspellings, the kidnappers asked for $20,000, about $480,000 in 2022 dollars, and warned the family not to contact the police. One note read in part, "You wil hav pay us befor you git him from us. An pay us a big cent to … if you regard his lif puts no one to search for him you money can fech him out alive an no other existin powers."

Charley Ross was never found. One of his alleged kidnappers died before he could reveal the boy's location. The website Heroes, Heroines & History says the warning "Don't take candy from strangers" derived from Charley's kidnapping. The packet of ransom notes sold for $20,000, the same amount as Charley's ransom.

This walk ends here. Cross the bridge for a West Philadelphia tour (pages 166 and 171), or go south to explore Fitler Square (page 40).

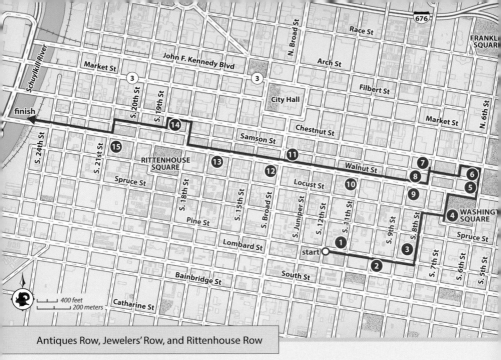

Antiques Row, Jewelers' Row, and Rittenhouse Row

Points of Interest

1. **Louis I. Kahn Park** S. 11th and Pine Sts., kahnpark.org

2. **M. Finkel & Daughter** 936 Pine St., 215-627-7797, samplings.com

3. **Pennsylvania Hospital** 800 Spruce St., 215-829-3000, pennmedicine.org

4. **Washington Square** 210 W. Washington Square, 215-965-2305, nps.gov/inde

5. **The Curtis Building** 601 Walnut St., 800-627-3999, keystonepropertygroup.com

6. **The Public Ledger Building** 149 S. Sixth St.

7. **Craftsman Row Saloon** 112 S. Eighth St., 215-923-0123, craftsmanrowsaloon.com

8. **Walnut Street Theatre** 825 Walnut St., 215-574-3550, walnutstreettheatre.org

9. **Wills Eye Hospital** 840 Walnut St., 215-928-3000, willseye.org

10. **The Forrest Theatre** 1114 Walnut St., 215-923-1515, forrest-theatre.com

11. **The Witherspoon Building** 1319–1323 Walnut St.

12. **Former Bellevue-Stratford Hotel (now The Bellevue Hotel)** 200 S. Broad St., 215-893-1234, bellevuephiladelphia.com

13. **Icon** 1616 Walnut St., 844-483-9141, icon1616.com

14. **Boyd's** 1818 Chestnut St., 215-564-9000, boydsphila.com

15. **First Presbyterian Church** 201 S. 21st St., 215-567-0532, fpcphila.org

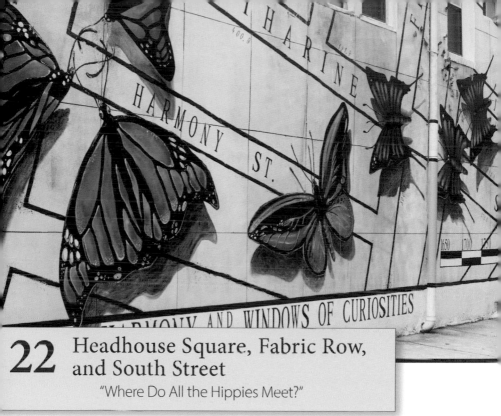

22 Headhouse Square, Fabric Row, and South Street

"Where Do All the Hippies Meet?"

Above. Conrad Booker's Harmony and the Windows of Curiosities *shows an early street map.*

BOUNDARIES: Pine St., Christian St., S. Second St., Schuylkill River
DISTANCE: 2 miles
DIFFICULTY: Easy
PARKING: This tour begins at S. Second and Lombard Streets. There is a private parking lot about a block away in the 200 block of Pine Street and abundant metered street parking.
PUBLIC TRANSIT: SEPTA's 40 bus stops nearby.

Part of William Penn's original street grid, South Street separates Center City from South Philadelphia. In 1963, R & B girl group The Orlons earned a gold record with "South Street," which included the lines "Where do all the hippies meet? South Street, South Street." In the 1960s and 1970s, the area was known for its bars, live-music venues, and the counterculture types who hung out there. In the late 1970s and early 1980s, South Street attracted punk rock fans.

The bohemian feel faded away in the 1990s as rents rose and funky boutiques gave way to chain stores and tourist traps. More recently the street seems to be undergoing another renaissance, with artists reclaiming gallery space and independent vegan and vegetarian food joints opening their doors.

Walk Description

Begin at South Second and Lombard Streets at the covered brick ❶ **Headhouse Square.** This former fire station was built in 1805 with a $1,000 donation from Joseph Witherill, whose Revolutionary War contribution was building new or converting old mills for the manufacture of gunpowder. The Headhouse leads to the New Market or The Shambles, an Old English term for a butcher stall. Founded in 1745 and still used today, this is the country's oldest surviving Colonial marketplace. The structure is typical of the rural English markets at the time, with parallel rows of brick pillars supporting a gabled roof.

Walk south through the Shambles, passing 401 S. Second Street, which belonged to John Ross, flag maker Betsy's uncle by marriage. George Washington reportedly visited for tea. The stretch between Lombard and South Streets underwent an overhaul in 2020 that removed parking spaces and added a brick path, picnic tables, and two maroon canopies.

Continue to South Street, the southern border of the original city. Up until the 1850s, criminals fleeing police needed only to cross to the south side of South Street to escape into Philadelphia County, writes Jim Murphy in *Real Philly History, Real Fast.* If officers wanted to continue the pursuit, they needed to contact the county sheriff. An 1854 decree made the boundaries of the city and county identical as it remains today. To the left is the Delaware River. Across the street, Head House Books (619 S. Second St.) is an independent store that encourages customers to "stay curious."

Turn right onto South Street, walking west. Rita's Italian Ice (239 South St.) is a local institution that grew into a national franchise. Philadelphia firefighter Bob Tumolo opened the first Rita's store in nearby Bensalem, Pennsylvania, in 1984, naming it after his wife. Rita's gives away free Italian ice on the first day of spring. The three most popular flavors are mango, cherry, and Swedish Fish.

Cross South Third Street. The Three Stooges's Larry Fine was born in the house that stood at 300 South Street as Louis Feinberg in 1902. In the accompanying mural, he plays the violin, as he did in many Stooges films, including 1936's *Disorder in the Court.* When Fine was a child, his forearm muscles were damaged by acid that his father, a jeweler, used to test gold. His parents had him take violin and boxing lessons to regain his strength.

Across the street, ❷ **Lorenzo and Sons Pizza** is known for the enormous slices it sells to lines of bar patrons in the wee hours of the morning. Experienced patrons know the staff can be a bit gruff;

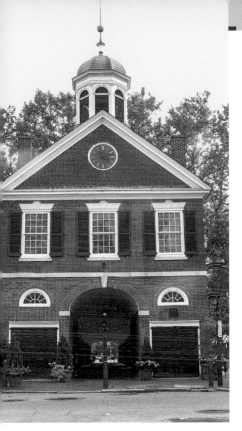

The Headhouse leads to an outdoor market formerly known as The Shambles.

special requests are not encouraged. For years, a sign boasted that this was a place "Where the Customer is Never Right." The restaurant's facade and three-story interior got a postfire face-lift in 2013. The tragedy also prompted owner Giuseppe Pulizzi to update his no-toppings policy: slices with toppings are now available on Tuesday until midnight. South Street Sushi or a Philly Taco is a slice of Lorenzo and Sons' pizza wrapped around a cheesesteak sandwich from nearby Jim's Steaks.

Continue to the ❸ **Theatre of Living Arts.** The concert venue opened in 1908 as a nickelodeon called the Crystal Palace with room for 500 people. The building has had various uses since, including as a movie theater, a repertory stage, and a nightclub. In 1987, concert company Live Nation Philadelphia purchased and rehabbed TLA, removing 75 pounds of rice that had been thrown at the screen during the weekly midnight viewings of *The Rocky Horror Picture Show*. In 2020, doctors from the University of Pennsylvania distributed more than 28,000 COVID-19 vaccination shots here.

Continue on South Street, stopping at South Fourth Street. Look right to see ❹ **Crash Bang Boom.** It was originally located about a block away and called Zipperhead. The legendary punk rock shop is mentioned in The Dead Milkmen's song "Punk Rock Girl." The store's former location at 407 South Street still bears an oversize painted zipper and giant ant sculptures climbing from the second floor to the roof. In 2022, local leaders announced the building would become the South Street Museum.

❺ **Jim's Steaks** often has a line snaking from its front door and down the block. Tourists often ask which of the city's two iconic cheesesteak joints is better, Pat's or Geno's. One faction of locals will always reply, "Jim's." Unlike Pat's and Geno's, Jim's has a full sandwich menu as well as indoor seating.

Across the street, MilkBoy (401 South St.) is a restaurant/bar venue. On the company's website, the FAQs include, "Do you guys have milkshakes?" The answer: "No, for the last time, no. Have a beer."

At South Fourth Street, turn left. Walk through Bainbridge Green, a shady stretch from South Third to South Fifth Streets, to reach ❻ **Famous 4th Street Delicatessen**. The Famous, in operation since 1923, is a city landmark and a popular Election Day gathering place for politicians and journalists since the 1970s. In 2010, President Barack Obama stopped by for a corned beef Reuben and potato pancakes, two of the deli's specialties. The deli has served as a movie backdrop. In the Oscar-winning 1993 film *Philadelphia,* Denzel Washington leaves the deli with a pastrami sandwich before agreeing to take on Tom Hanks's lawsuit.

If ordering a sandwich, be warned: They are called overstuffed for a reason—one sandwich can easily feed two or three diners. The deli is also known for its chocolate chip cookies, which are also available at its Reading Terminal Market location.

Continue south on Fabric Row, the one-time center of the city's Eastern European Jewish community's commercial life, known as Der Ferder ("the fourth" in Yiddish). Textile dealers began selling goods here—either in storefronts or with pushcarts—at the beginning of the 20th century. Pushcarts were outlawed in the 1950s, and many of the textile shops closed in the following decades. The area's revitalization began in the early 2000s.

❼ **Brickbat Books** is an independent store. When its owner was diagnosed with brain cancer in 2017, more than a dozen locals rearranged their lives to work free shifts in the store. Some did so for more than two years.

Continue to Fulton Street. ❽ *Harmony and the Windows of Curiosities* is the work of neighborhood resident Conrad Booker. The map is from 1865 and includes a recently uncovered nearby African American cemetery.

At Christian Street, turn right. ❾ **Settlement Music School** was founded in 1908 by two women offering immigrant children piano lessons for a nickel. It now has six locations. Among the well-known musicians who studied here are Chubby Checker and Mario Lanza. Albert Einstein was a member of the school's advisory board.

Continue to South Fifth Street and turn right. While walking through this residential stretch, note the many ways residents personalize their properties, including flowers, door decor, outdoor furniture, and front window displays.

Continue to South Street and turn left. ❿ **Philadelphia's Magic Gardens** is the next stop. To get an idea of what's coming, look for artist Isaiah Zagar's work—brightly colored mosaics made of tile and cut mirror—along this stretch. The nearby Schell Street alley is covered with his works. The door at 824–826 South Street features his self-portrait.

Zagar began work on his half-block-long public art project near his studio in 1994 and continues to expand it. In 2002, the owner of some of the lots called for the art to be removed and the lots sold. After a two-year legal battle and help from the local community, Philadelphia's Magic Gardens was incorporated as a nonprofit that hosts workshops, concerts, and other events. Visitors can enter the indoor art galleries for a small charge.

Continue on South Street. Just past South 12th Street is a historical marker for the Standard Theatre. African American businessman John T. Gibson purchased the property in 1914 to offer "High Class and Meritorious Vaudeville" shows and music, according to explorepahistory.com. It was a tough business for African Americans: in 1927, Duke Ellington and his band were playing the Standard when the white owner of New York's Cotton Club decided he wanted Ellington to play at his club. A stranger approached the Standard's theater manager to ask him to let the band go, saying, "Be big. Or you'll be dead." Still, the Standard did well. It appealed to both black and white audiences, making it a "black-and-tans."

Continue to ⑪ *The Atlas of Tomorrow: A Device for Philosophical Reflection*, the city's first interactive mural, which challenges viewers to ask a question and then spin a 6-foot dial. The spinner stops at a number corresponding with a story on the bottom of the mural, all of which are modified from *The I Ching*, one of the world's oldest books of wisdom. The person can then interpret the message as desired. The art itself is made from thousands of fingerprints.

Artist Isaiah Zagar has adorned the city with his mosaics. Philadelphia's Magic Gardens showcases his most impressive work.

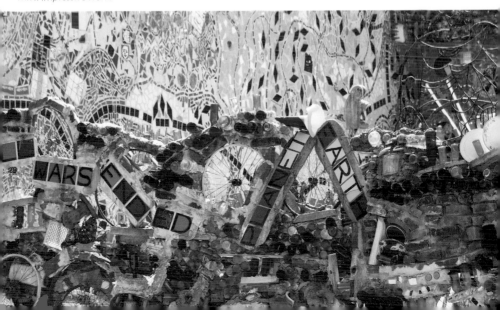

Cross South Broad Street. **12** *Billiards: A Tribute to Edward "Chick" Davis* shows two men playing pool, including one of the sport's greatest, Willie Mosconi (center), a South Philadelphian who picked up a cue at age 6. Between 1941 and 1957, he won 15 straight world championships. During a two-day exhibition in Ohio in the 1950s, he won a record 526 straight games. In the mural he holds one of his designer cues made by Russian-born craftsman George Balabushka, whose cues are considered the Stradivariuses of the billiards world. Mosconi had several, all inlaid with mother-of-pearl.

The other player is Edward "Chick" Davis, who learned to play billiards at the first YMCA open to African Americans. Since African Americans were barred from playing in pool halls, Davis honed his skills after hours, eventually competing against Mosconi. With his winnings, Davis opened pool halls in the city, including the one where this mural is painted.

13 *Legendary,* on the wall of the now-closed World Communications Charter School, is a tribute to The Roots, the Grammy Award–winning, Philadelphia-born band now known as the house band for *The Tonight Show Starring Jimmy Fallon.* In the early 1990s, the musicians were buskers collecting change from passersby. The mural is a few blocks from the Philadelphia High School for the Creative and Performing Arts, the band's founder's alma mater.

This block was also the location of Mae Reeves' original hat shop. Reeves was one of the first African American women to own a business in the city, opening Mae's Millinery Shop in 1940. Her clients included Lena Horne, Marian Anderson, and Ella Fitzgerald. Two rooms from the shop have been re-created in the National Museum of African American History and Culture.

Continue west, passing **14** **Bob & Barbara's Lounge,** a local institution serving its Citywide Special—a can of Pabst Blue Ribbon and a shot of Jim Beam—since 1969.

The now-closed **15** **Royal Theater,** built in 1919, showcased well-known performers including Billie Holiday, Cab Calloway, and Pearl Bailey. A mural on the facade shows the building when it was a hub of African American life. In the 1930s, the theater added movies, with one sign declaring it "America's Finest Colored Photoplayhouse." It closed in 1970.

This walk ends here. For the Rittenhouse Square tour (page 33), continue to South 18th Street and turn right.

Points of Interest

1 **Headhouse Square and The Shambles** Pine and South Second Sts., southstreet.com

2 **Lorenzo and Sons Pizza** 305 South St., 215-800-1942, facebook.com/LorenzoAndSonsPizza

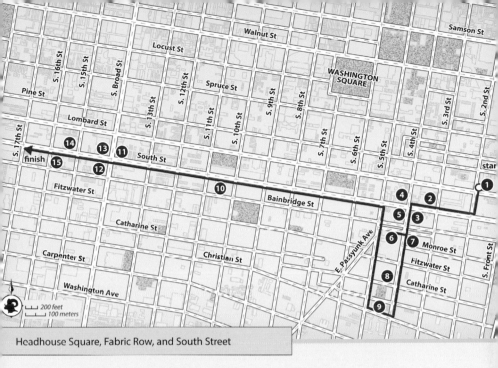

Headhouse Square, Fabric Row, and South Street

3 **Theatre of Living Arts** 334 South St., 215 922 1011, venue.tlaphilly.com

4 **Crash Bang Boom** 528 S. Fourth St., 215-928-1123, crashbangboomonline.com

5 **Jim's Steaks** 400 South St., 215-928-1911, jimssouthstreet.com

6 **Famous 4th Street Delicatessen** 700 S. Fourth St., 215-922-3274, famous4thstreetdelicatessen.com

7 **Brickbat Books** 709 S. Fourth St., 215-592-1207, brickbatbooks.blogspot.com

8 **Harmony and the Windows of Curiosities** 770 S. Fourth St. Mural Arts Philadelphia, 215-685-0750, muralarts.org

9 **Settlement Music School** 416 Queen St., 215-320-2601, settlementmusic.org

10 **Philadelphia's Magic Gardens** 1020 South St., 215-733-0390, phillymagicgardens.org

11 **The Atlas of Tomorrow: A Device for Philosophical Reflection** South and Juniper Sts. Mural Arts Philadelphia, 215-685-0750, muralarts.org

12 **Billiards: A Tribute to Edward "Chick" Davis** 1412 South St.

13 **Legendary** 512 S. Broad St. Mural Arts Philadelphia, 215-685-0750, muralarts.org

14 **Bob & Barbara's Lounge** 1509 South St., 215-545-4511, bobandbarbaras.com

15 **Former Royal Theater** 1536 South St.

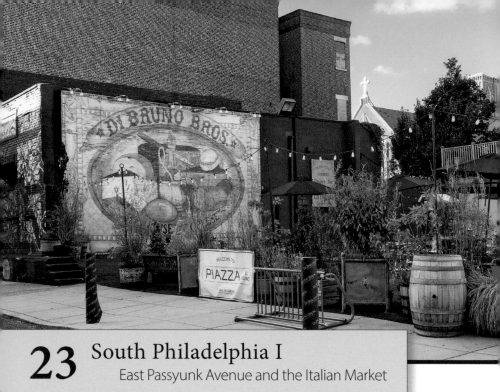

23 South Philadelphia I
East Passyunk Avenue and the Italian Market

Above: Brothers Danny and Joe Di Bruno opened their eponymous shop in 1939.

BOUNDARIES: Broad St., S. Seventh St., Bainbridge St., Passyunk Ave.
DISTANCE: 2 miles
DIFFICULTY: Easy
PARKING: Metered street parking and pay lots are available.
PUBLIC TRANSIT: SEPTA's Broad Street line subway, at Tasker Ave., is about 2 blocks from the start of this walk. Buses that cross E. Passyunk Ave. include the 4, 23, and 29. Buses that stop within a few blocks include the 2, 37, 47, and 47m.

Italian immigrants began settling here as early as the 1700s, but it was the mass migrations at the end of the 1800s and early 1900s that established this area as the city's Little Italy. (No one ever calls it that, though.) The outdoor fruit and vegetable market—which looks little changed since Rocky Balboa ran through it in the 1970s—is often called the Italian Market, although the majority of businesses are no longer owned by Italian Americans.

This walk features a section of Italian American—or formerly Italian American—South Philadelphia, including the nation's first Italian American Catholic church, the first Italian mutual aid society, and the city's first Italian restaurant. Enjoy a *passeggiata,* an Italian term for a leisurely stroll.

Walk Description

Begin at South Broad Street and East Passyunk Avenue, following East Passyunk Avenue northeast. This was originally a Native American trail, the name coming from the word *pachsegink,* which means "in the valley" or "a place of sleep." Locals pronounce it "PASH-yunk" or "PASS-yunk." Manhole covers feature a native man wearing a feathered headdress.

Follow the road as it curves left. At Mifflin Street, turn right. Cross South 13th Street. The pen-and-ink vinyl panels of *East Passyunk—Crossing through the Ages* (South 13th and Mifflin Sts.) were installed on this closed transportation substation in 2015.

Turn around and walk to the median park. The bronze statue honors Joey Giardello, a former world middleweight boxing champion who trained nearby. The 1999 movie *The Hurricane* includes Giardello's 1964 middleweight title match against Rubin Carter. Giardello won by unanimous decision, but the movie implied Carter should have been the victor. Giardello sued the filmmakers, winning an undisclosed settlement and the agreement that the DVD version of the film would include commentary calling Giardello a great fighter.

Continue on East Passyunk. The ❶ **History of Italian Immigration Museum** features the stories of local Italian American families. Inscribed on its sidewalk are the names of museum donors.

In the 1930s, a tailor shop on this block was the unofficial headquarters of the Philadelphia Poison Ring. Led by cousins Paul Petrillo, a tailor, and Herman Petrillo, a spaghetti salesman, the gang killed dozens of men, usually with arsenic, then collected thousands of dollars in insurance money. In some cases, the men's wives were willing accomplices. Rose Carina was thought to have killed five husbands. When she was arrested in 1939, the Associated Press reported, she "was given an ovation by the other women inmates at Moyamensing Prison."

In others instances, the widows were duped, given a special powder and told it was a love potion or an elixir that would erase their husbands' bad habits. At least 25 people were arrested for their involvement in the ring. The actual number of victims is unknown, although news articles reported at least 100 deaths. The case drew national attention. Another 1939 AP article refers to "Philadelphia's phantasmagoria of poison-for-profit," calling the crimes "the greatest mass murder plot in American history."

A passeggiata note: Stargazy (1838 E. Passyunk) serves British meat pies, specializing in one with jellied eels—they're easy to hold while walking.

Continue walking. Anna and Pasquale Scioli opened their eponymous tailoring shop at 1744 E. Passyunk soon after emigrating from Italy in 1967. Their business soon became known as the "Tailor to the Stars," custom fitting suits for city politicians, high-powered lawyers, and professional athletes on and off the field. But those in need of a hem need not be intimidated: The Sciolis serve regular folks, too, sending customers of all backgrounds off with a "Take it eeze!"

2 **Marra's Italian Restaurant,** opened by Neapolitan immigrants Chiarina and Salvatore Marra in the 1920s, is still family owned and using the oven Salvatore built with bricks from Mount Vesuvius. Legend says Frank Sinatra was nicknamed Ol' Blue Eyes by a waitress who saw him and swooned, "Oh my God, those beautiful blue eyes."

Marra's is what locals consider a red gravy or red sauce restaurant. Some background: Some Northeastern Italian Americans refer to that tomato-based, meat-infused, garlic-enhanced, basil-accented deliciousness on spaghetti as gravy. This confused non-Italians who believe gravy is the brown liquid served on Thanksgiving. In kindness to the confused, those of Italian descent sometimes put the word *red* before gravy. A red-gravy or red-sauce restaurant is one specializing in basics, such as spaghetti and meatballs, lasagna, and manicotti. Marra's serves pizza, but don't expect that at all red-gravy restaurants.

Continue on East Passyunk Avenue. Two murals flank the lot at 1600 E. Passyunk. On the right, *History of Passyunk* shows the changing street scenes from the area's 125 years.

The other is somewhat puzzling. **3** *Pathology of Devotion* "appears to depict a World War II–era submariner using a periscope to spy on actor Robin Williams. Curiously, Williams is holding a rosary," a 2008 *Philadelphia Inquirer* article concluded. The same article quoted a Mural Arts Philadelphia spokeswoman saying the intent was to represent the intersection of science and religion. (The guy in the puffy shirt is a priest hearing confession.)

Continue, crossing Tasker Street. **4** **The Singing Fountain** is a popular pocket park with speakers hidden around the square that allow the fountain to "sing." Locals enjoy lounging on benches or playing chess while visitors kill time before dinner reservations.

The Acme supermarket (1400 E. Passyunk) is built on the former site of Moyamensing Prison, also called Moko or the Philadelphia County Prison. The country's first serial killer, H. H. Holmes, was put to death by hanging here in 1896. Edgar Allan Poe and Al Capone each spent a night. Some members of the Philadelphia Poison Ring were also held here.

Continue on East Passyunk Avenue. At Wharton Street, the community garden and murals replaced an empty lot holding dumpsters in 2011. There was a minor mural controversy because of the panel with "Passyunk's Finest Pears." Locals griped that pears had nothing to do with

South Philadelphia. The beleaguered artist said he'd painted pears because it started with *P*, like Passyunk. The white-haired man is Harry Olivieri, a founder of nearby Pat's King of Steaks.

Cross Wharton Street. Welcome to Cheesesteak Vegas, home to the city's best-known cheesesteak shops: ❺ **Pat's King of Steaks** and ❻ **Geno's Steaks.** Pat's says they invented the cheesesteak in 1930. Geno's opened in 1966.

The perpetual question from cheesesteak-seeking out-of-towners is, "Pat's or Geno's?" This book takes no stand, but be warned: Philadelphians take cheesesteaks seriously, so it's best to know how to order before reaching the counter. Here's some guidance:

1. Decide which type of cheese is desired. The options are Cheez Whiz (traditional choice), American (still OK), or provolone (acceptable). To stray is to be mocked: In 2003, Democratic presidential candidate John Kerry asked for Swiss, appalling locals. Once schooled and given a sandwich dripping with processed cheese sauce, Kerry "made matters worse by delicately nibbling at it as if it were tea toast," *The Philadelphia Inquirer* reported.

2. Decide on onions. If desired, remember the word *with*. If no, remember the word *without*.

3. Now order. Example: To get one cheesesteak with Cheez Whiz and onions, and another with American cheese but no onions, say, "I'll have a Whiz with and an American without."

Good luck.

At Ninth Street, turn left. ❼ **Capitolo Playground,** established in 1839, is on the former site of Lafayette Cemetery, where more than 47,000 people, including Civil War veterans, were interred. In the 1940s, the city reclaimed the land and hired a company to remove the dead and rebury them respectfully. In 1988, construction workers building a suburban mall stumbled upon 30 trenches filled with hundreds of caskets from Lafayette Cemetery. *The Melting Pot*, wrapped around the playground's main building, features the faces of neighborhood residents.

Continue on South Ninth Street. Immigrants from the Mexican state of Puebla began settling here en masse in the 1980s and own many businesses here. This community hosts El Carnaval de Puebla en Filadelfia, one of the nation's largest Cinco de Mayo celebrations.

Cross Washington Avenue. The ❽ **9th Street Italian Market** was featured in the *Rocky* movies. In the first, filmed in 1976, the then-unknown Sylvester Stallone ran through the market without drawing much attention. That memorable scene when a vendor throws Rocky an orange?

Not scripted. The vendor later said he just wanted to toss something to the dirty guy in the gray sweat suit. It made the movie.

The 9th Street market has changed a lot since that movie hit the theaters. It is no longer dominated by Italian vendors. Mexican and Vietnamese merchants have a strong presence. That's why some people have taken "Italian" out of the name, calling it the South 9th Street Curb Market.

But in other ways, the market seems timeless: Vendors still warm themselves via trash-can fires in the winter. Fruits and vegetables are sold in bulk and for cheap.

Villa Di Roma (936 S. Ninth St.) is a red-gravy joint offering no-frills but solid food and sassy service. Epiphany "Pip" De Luca's father purchased the restaurant and a neighboring bar in the 1960s. One of Pip's first jobs was bartending. In a 2014 interview with the *Philadelphia Inquirer*, he described opening the bar on Mondays at 7 a.m.: "Monday is the day of rest on Ninth Street, so all the merchants would gather here around 7:30 in the morning and talk about the business they'd done during the week. The deals they made that turned out to be good, the deals they made that turned out lousy. They'd come in and drink their shots and beers, their coffee and anisette. And smoke, and play their numbers with the numbers writers."

Continue north. **9 Di Bruno Bros.** was a grocery store opened by brothers Danny and Joe Di Bruno in 1939. In 1965, facing stiff competition from supermarkets, they reinvented themselves as a specialty shop.

10 Claudio's Specialty Foods, opened by Italian immigrants Salvatrice and Claudio Auriemma Sr. in the 1950s, has cheeses taller than the average-size American woman hanging from the ceiling.

At Christian Street, turn left. Christopher Columbus Charter School (916 Christian St.) was Christian Street Hospital, the first Civil War Army hospital. Doctors at this 220-bed facility pioneered treatments for nerve disorders and gunshot wounds. One coined the term *phantom limb* to describe the sensation amputees had.

Continue west, passing St. Paul Church (923 Christian St.). Cross South 10th Street. **11 Isgro** Italian bakery, a neighborhood mainstay since 1904, is known for its cannoli. Framed letters on the wall include a thank you from tenor Luciano Pavarotti, who enjoyed an Isgro's birthday cake.

Turn around. At South 10th Street, turn left. **12 Dante & Luigi's,** opened in 1899, offers red-gravy dishes and more modern fare. Originally called Corona di Ferro, this was a destination for Italian immigrants, who arrived at the docks with the restaurant's name written on a piece of paper pinned to their lapel. The workers lived in rooms upstairs while working as cooks and waiters. President Joe Biden's family has long had an account here.

The restaurant was also the site of an attempted mob hit. In 1989, a man wearing a Batman mask entered the restaurant and shot Nicky Scarfo Jr. eight times in the neck, arms, and torso. Scarfo, son of Philadelphia mob boss Nicky Scarfo, survived. Formerly known as "Little Nicky," Scarfo was dubbed "Lucky Nicky" after the shooting.

At Fitzwater Street, turn right. ⓭ **Sam's Morning Glory Diner** is another breakfast/lunch favorite. (Be prepared: it's cash only.)

Continue on Fitzwater to South Ninth Street. ⓮ **Palumbo Playground and Recreation Center** was once Ronaldson Cemetery, a nonreligious burial space, in the 1820s. More than 13,000 people were interred here. In the 1950s, the city reclaimed the land, moving the dead to a mass grave in northeast Philadelphia. (A few "celebrity" dead—including several Revolutionary War soldiers—were relocated to Old Swedes Church's cemetery.)

At South Ninth Street, turn right. At ⓯ **Sarcone's Bakery,** lines snake down the street on weekends and before holidays.

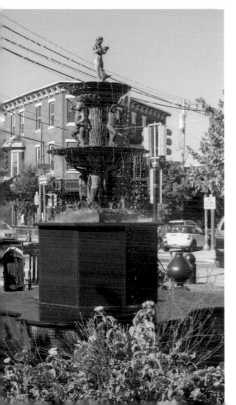

Locals and guests enjoy the Singing Fountain.

Continue south. ⓰ **Ralph's** is a family-run red-gravy restaurant in business since 1900. Theodore Roosevelt dined here, according to their website, and President Biden visited frequently when he represented Delaware in the US Senate.

At Catharine Street, turn left. Walk to South Eighth Street. Make a right, then a quick left to continue on Catharine Street. *Autumn Revisited* is on the side of ⓱ **Samuel S. Fleisher Art Memorial,** an arts center offering tuition-free lessons and low-cost workshops to children and adults. In the 1890s, Samuel Fleisher became vice president of the yarn company founded by his German Jewish immigrant parents. At his sister's suggestion, he began offering free art classes to his workers' children. When he died in 1944, his fortune was left in trust to perpetuate these classes. The center welcomes more than 6,000 students annually.

Stop at South Seventh Street. Italian American singers Bobby Rydell—born Roberto Ridarelli—and Mario Lanza attended elementary school at the former St. Mary Magdalen de Pazzi Elementary School (825 S. Seventh St.), now condos. Lanza was born in a home at 636 Christian Street.

Across South Seventh Street is neighborhood staple ⓲ **John's Water Ice**, opened by Sicilian immigrants in 1945. It offers fruit-flavored ice similar to Italian ice, but it's softer with a less concentrated flavor. The traditional offerings are lemon, chocolate, and cherry, but John's has been known to surprise people with banana or mango. President Obama ordered lemon during his 2011 visit.

Continue south, crossing Christian Street. Banca Calabrese (638 Christian St.) opened in 1902 to serve the banking needs of Italian immigrants. It was one of many banks that tailored services to a specific ethnic group. This is now a residential building.

At Montrose Street, turn right. ⓳ **St. Mary Magdalen de Pazzi** is the first Italian American Catholic parish in the country. Mario Lanza allegedly sang in the choir here.

This walk ends here. Continue two blocks on Montrose Street to return to the Italian Market.

Points of Interest

❶ History of Italian Immigration Museum 1834 E. Passyunk Ave., 215-334-8882, filitaliainternational.com

❷ Marra's Italian Restaurant 1734 E. Passyunk Ave., 215-463-9249, marrasone.com

❸ *Pathology of Devotion* 1644 E. Passyunk Ave.

❹ The Singing Fountain S. 11th St. and E. Passyunk Ave.

❺ Pat's King of Steaks 1237 E. Passyunk Ave., 215-468-1546, patskingofsteaks.com

❻ Geno's Steaks 1219 S. Ninth St., 215-389-0659, genosteaks.com

❼ Capitolo Playground 900 Federal St., 215-685-1883

❽ 9th Street Italian Market 215-278-2903, italianmarketphilly.org

❾ Di Bruno Bros. 930 S. Ninth St., 215-922-2876, dibruno.com

❿ Claudio's Specialty Foods 924 S. Ninth St., 215-627-1873, claudiofood.com

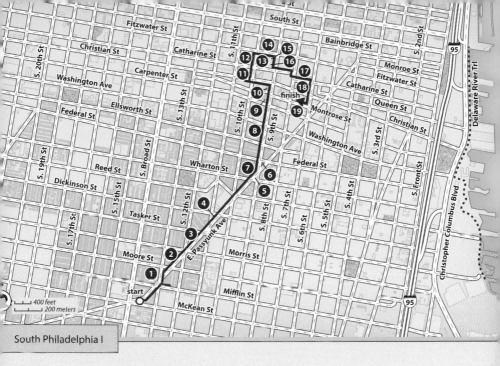

11   **Isgro**   1009 Christian St., 215-923-3092, isgropastries.com

12   **Dante & Luigi's**   762 S. 10th St., 215-922-9501, danteandluigis.com

13   **Sam's Morning Glory Diner**   735 S. 10th St., 215-413-3999, facebook.com/MorningGloryDiner

14   **Palumbo Playground and Recreation Center**   700 S. Ninth St., 215-592-6007, palumborec.org

15   **Sarcone's Bakery**   758 S. Ninth St., 215-922-0445, sarconesbakery.com

16   **Ralph's**   760 S. Ninth St., 215-627-6011, ralphsrestaurant.com

17   **Samuel S. Fleisher Art Memorial**   719 Catharine St., 215-922-3456, fleisher.org

18   **John's Water Ice**   701 Christian St., 215-925-6955, johnswaterice.com

19   **St. Mary Magdalen de Pazzi**   712 Montrose St., stpaulparish.net

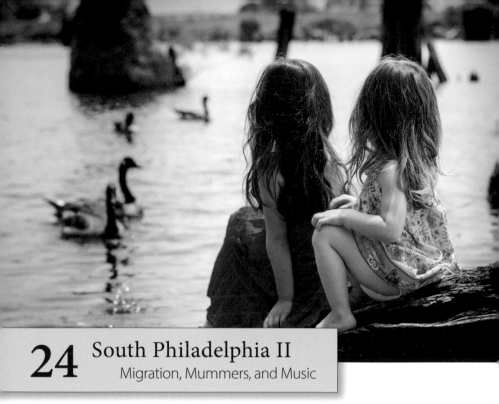

Above: Washington Avenue Green, a park on the Delaware River, is a peaceful reprieve.

BOUNDARIES: Bainbridge St., Washington Ave., Schuylkill River, S. 11th St.
DISTANCE: 3.6 miles
DIFFICULTY: Easy
PARKING: There is 2-hour street parking available here, as well as an outdoor pay lot.
PUBLIC TRANSIT: SEPTA bus stops dot the area where this tour begins, including the 21 to Penn's Landing, the 40 to S. Second and Lombard Sts., or the 64 to Washington Ave. and Columbus Blvd.

South Philadelphia was "the city's first ethnic ghetto," Murray Dubin writes in *South Philadelphia: Mummers, Memories, and the Melrose Diner*, and it continues to attract immigrants from throughout the world, with those from Mexico and Southeast Asia among the most recent to settle here.

Walk Description

Begin at Front and Chestnut Streets, where the Old City tour (page 98) ended. ❶ **The Irish Memorial** honors the millions who died during Ireland's Potato Famine in the mid-1800s and the survivors who emigrated to England, Australia, Canada, and the United States. This 30-foot-long sculpture in the round was commissioned for the famine's 150th anniversary. The engraved poem by Peter Quinn begins, "The hunger ended/but it never went away/It was there in silent memories,/From one generation,/to the next. . . ."

Next to the memorial is the *Commemoration of Scottish Immigration to America,* the first national memorial acknowledging the contributions of Scottish immigrants. It was installed in 2011 and paid for by the St. Andrew's Society of Philadelphia, an organization named for Scotland's patron saint and founded in 1747 by Scots seeking to help newly arriving countrymen.

Follow the right path to Front Street. A marker remembers the Tun Tavern, where the St. Andrew's Society originated.

At Front Street, turn left. At left is the Delaware River and the site where, in 1855, an enslaved woman named Jane Johnson and her sons escaped with help from local abolitionists who were then arrested and accused of kidnapping the family. Johnson returned to the city to speak on their behalf, saying she left on her own, "I don't want to go back . . . I'd sooner die than go back."

At Dock Street, the ❷ **Philadelphia Korean War Memorial** at Penn's Landing, dedicated in 2001, honors the more than 600 men from the Philadelphia area who died in the conflict.

At Dock Street, turn left. At Columbus Boulevard, turn right, passing Thomas Foglietta Plaza, named for a former city council member who served in the US House of Representatives and later as the US ambassador to Italy.

Continue to the ❸ **Philadelphia Vietnam Veterans Memorial,** which honors the more than 650 American soldiers killed in Vietnam who said Philadelphia was their home of record. In 2016, two names—Master Sergeants George Wilson and Francis Corcoran—were added to the wall. Corcoran's widow attended the dedication.

Walk through the plaza, exiting via the path to the left of the statue of a soldier. Turn left, continuing on Front Street. Crossing South Street, at left is *Stroll,* a 1995 sculpture featuring three large metal figures crossing the highway overpass. A 2013 *Philadelphia* article described it thusly: "The three figures—strolling hand-in-hand to South Street to buy some novelty t-shirts and bongs, no doubt—have weird, bowling-pin shaped heads and a leg-to-torso ratio not found in any humans I've ever seen." The sculpture's hidden meaning, the article said, is that "One day, metal monsters will destroy us all."

Continue south, passing the former home of US naval officer Stephen Decatur, which is now a Veterans of Foreign Wars chapter. Decatur became a national hero in 1803 when the USS *Philadelphia* was captured by pirates in Tripoli. He and his crew sailed the harbor disguised as tradesmen and destroyed the ship so America's enemies could not use it. British admiral Horatio Lord Nelson called this "the most bold and daring act of the age."

At Kenilworth Street, turn right. At South Second Street, turn left. At Monroe Street, turn right. Men often played cards after enjoying a shvitz at Kratchman's Bathhouses, which once stood at 313–321 Monroe Street. The only remnant is a small sign designating BATH HOUSE COURT.

Continue west to South Fourth Street and Fabric Row. In the early 1900s, Jewish merchants sold fabric from pushcarts here. The neighborhood has changed, but more than half a dozen fabric businesses remain.

Continue straight. The Art Deco ❹ **Meredith Elementary School**, built in 1931, is named for William M. Meredith, a Philadelphia attorney who served as President Zachary Taylor's Treasury Secretary. The school's mural is *CornerSmile/Peace Through Imagination,* named for the oversize lips emerging from the corner.

Walk one block south on Fifth Street. Turn right on Fitzwater Street. At Passyunk Avenue, turn right. At Fitzwater Street, turn left.

❺ **Cianfrani Park** is named for late politician Henry "Buddy" Cianfrani's mother. Cianfrani, a beloved son of South Philly, saw his star rise, then fall, then rise again. A World War II veteran, Cianfrani was a state senator when convicted on federal racketeering and mail fraud charges for having fake employees on his payroll. After leaving jail, he became a popular political adviser.

The Southwark Soup Society (833 Fitzwater St.) was founded in 1805 as a charity dedicated to providing the "deserving poor" with hot meals and free coal during the winter.

At South Eighth Street, turn right. At Bainbridge Street, turn left. ❻ **The Church of the Crucifixion** opened in 1846 and was one of the city's first integrated congregations in "the poorest and most violent section of what was to become South Philadelphia," its website says. Marian Anderson made her singing debut here. As she later recounted, "One day when I was on my way to the grocery store to buy something for my mother, my eyes caught sight of a small handbill lying on the street. I picked it up, and there in a corner was my picture with my name under it. 'Come hear the baby contralto, 10 years old,' it said. I was actually 8. What excitement!" The church was closed for decades, reopening in 2021 with a focus on the Hispanic population.

Ahead on Bainbridge Street, the Institute for Colored Youth once occupied the residential building at 915 Bainbridge. It was funded by a Quaker philanthropist who wanted a school "to instruct

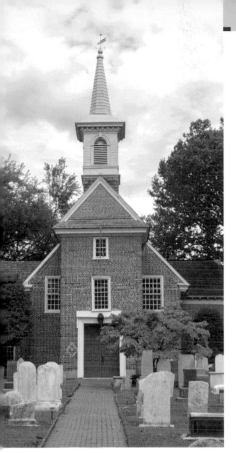

Gloria Dei Church, also known as Old Swedes,' was built around 1700.

the descendants of the African Race in school learning, in the various branches of the mechanic Arts, trades and Agriculture, in order to prepare and fit and qualify them to act as teachers."

Continue on Bainbridge Street, passing David Guinn's *Crystal Snowscape,* at South 10th Street. Poet Frances Ellen Watkins Harper lived at 1006 Bainbridge Street from 1870 until her death in 1911. She also wrote for antislavery newspapers. Some call her the mother of African American journalism.

Continue to South 11th Street and turn left. The Academy at Palumbo (1100 Catharine St.) was designed in 1920 by Irwin T. Catharine, the Meredith School architect. One innovation was adding a cafeteria so children didn't need to go home for lunch. Hidden City Philadelphia published a 1925 interview in which Catharine talked about replacing wooden partitions in bathrooms with white marble: "There is something in the nature of every boy which makes him want to carve his initial or whole name in a wall. If he isn't clever enough with his pocketknife, he writes his name. White marble partitions and walls make it impossible for him to use his knife." The website notes, "Sadly, Catharine could not foresee the effect that Sharpie markers would have on his marble."

Turn left on Catharine Street, passing Dante & Luigi's, one of the country's oldest family-owned Italian restaurants.

Frank Palumbo's Cabaret Restaurant once stood at 824–30 Catharine Street, where a drugstore is now. Palumbo said, "If I stop giving, I stop living." Actor-singer Mario Lanza, born and raised a few blocks from here, once said Palumbo was one of the city's unsung heroes. Sinatra was a frequent visitor to the club, where notables, including Jimmy Durante, Louis Prima, and Louis Armstrong, performed.

Continue to Darien Street and turn right. At Christian Street, turn left. For more than 125 years, the building housing **❼ Fiorella** was a butcher shop. In 2020, chef Marc Vetri converted the property into a casual pasta restaurant.

Continue to South Eighth Street. A marker near *Moonlit Landscape* (737 Christian St.) notes that the musically gifted Giannini Family lived and operated an Italian opera theater nearby. The Gianninis were opera stars: Father Feruccio was a tenor, mother Antoinetta a violinist, daughter Dusolina a soprano, and son Vittorio a composer.

Continue on Christian Street, passing the multifamily building at 636 Christian Street that in 2018 replaced Mario Lanza's home and birthplace. At South Sixth Street, turn left. At Queen Street, turn right. **❽ Weccacoe Playground** has been a play space for children for more than a century. During a 2013 renovation, workers found the tombstone of Amelia Brown, who died in 1819 at age 26. Further investigation uncovered the city's first private African American cemetery, Bethel Burying Ground. About 5,000 members of Mother Bethel African Methodist Church were interred here between 1810 and 1865. In 2021, city leaders announced plans to build a memorial at the site.

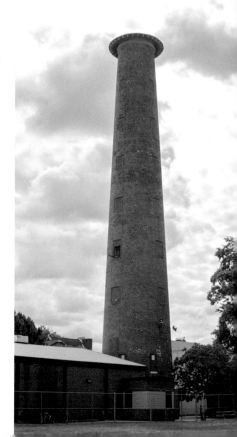

Sparks Shot Tower was the first shot manufacturing facility in the county.

Continue on Queen Street. Mario Lanza Park, on Queen Street between South Second and Third Streets, is named after the actor/singer born Alfred Cocozza just blocks away. Lanza did odd jobs to afford voice lessons. His stage name comes from his mother, Italian-born Maria Lanza.

Across the street is **❾ St. Philip Neri Church.** In 1844, an anti-Catholic mob attacked Irish American homes and Roman Catholic churches, killing at least 20 people and destroying two churches and a convent. St. Philip Neri survived because state militia guarded it. The parish today includes the neighborhood's original Polish church, **❿ St. Stanislaus Church,** named for Poland's patron saint and founded in the 1890s. Polish immigrants arriving at Washington Avenue Immigration Station "only had to walk across Delaware Avenue to find themselves not only in the new land of opportunity, but in a neighborhood where there was a church and school named after the patron saint of their homeland," according to the Polish American Cultural Center's website.

At South Second Street, turn right. At Carpenter Street, turn left. Signage showcases the city's love of replacing the letter *f* with *ph* to Philafy words. This sign advises drivers to proceed "CarePhilly."

Sparks Shot Tower (101–31 Carpenter St.) was the first shot manufacturing facility in the country, built in 1808. Ammunition was made by dropping dollops of hot lead from the top of the 142-foot tower through a copper sieve into water below. Previously, projectiles were imported from Britain. The tower became a city recreation center in 1913.

Continue to Front Street and turn left. At Christian Street, turn right. **⓫ Gloria Dei (Old Swedes') Episcopal Church** was built in 1698, making it the oldest church in the city. It has been in continuous use for more than 300 years, first by Swedish Lutherans, then as Episcopalians. One 18th-century pastor wrote that his New Jersey faithful could not boat across the river in winter without being "in gravous peril from floating ice," which "sometimes breaks large boats right in two," writes Jim Murphy in *Real Philly History, Real Fast*. Betsy Ross married her second husband, Joseph Ashburn, at Old Swedes in 1777. He was killed in the Revolutionary War. (Her first husband died that way too.)

Continue to Washington Avenue. Cross Columbus Boulevard. Follow the trail to Washington Avenue Green (1301 S. Columbus Blvd.), between the Coast Guard building and the union facility. Between 1873 and 1915, more than 1 million European immigrants passed through Washington Avenue Immigration Station, called Philadelphia's Ellis Island. The Southwark Historical Society says one room was called "the altar," as some single women weren't allowed to disembark until they wed.

The station was torn down in 1915. This was wasted land for almost a century until the Delaware River Waterfront Corporation revitalized the pier. *Land Buoy*, the 55-foot-tall spire topped with a blue light offers a great view.

Return to Columbus Boulevard, cross the road, and follow Washington Avenue to *Summary of Mummery* under the I-95 overpass, at 37 Washington Avenue. The Mummers Museum describes mummery thusly: "Mummers are people who belong to one of five types of clubs that participate in the annual New Year's Day parade. One group is composed of musicians who compete annually for the title of best string band. The others wear costumes, some fancy and some plain, and perform dance routines. Generations of families often walk together."

The first city-sponsored parade was in 1901, making it the country's oldest continuous folk parade. Today's parade is associated with first-class musicians—a good thing—and, unfortunately, excessive drinking. Still, that, too, seems to be traditional, as mummers once went door-to-door chanting, "Here we stand before your door/As we stood the year before/Give us whisky, give us gin/Open the door and let us in."

Continue west. **⑫ The Mummers Museum** opened in 1976 as part of the country's bicentennial celebration. The museum's website has a constant countdown measuring the weeks, days, hours, minutes, and seconds until the next January 1 parade. This stretch of South Second Street—called Two Street by Mummers—is the epicenter of Mummer life.

Pass Jefferson Square Park (Washington Ave. between S. Third and S. Fifth Sts.). Laid out in the early 1800s, the park was a Union Army camp during the Civil War.

End this tour at the corner of South Fifth Street. In the 1700s, this was Walnut Grove, a mansion belonging to merchant Joseph Wharton, a man with such a regal bearing that some called him "Duke Wharton." (No relation to the Joseph Wharton who founded the University of Pennsylvania's Wharton School of Business in 1881.)

During the Revolutionary War, the British Army occupied Philadelphia from September 1777 to June 1778. In April 1778, British officers organized a farewell party for General William Howe, who had resigned and was returning to England. They called it the "Meschianza," derived from the Italian word for medley.

More than 400 guests indulged in the decadent celebration, which included a Delaware River regatta carrying VIPs from what is now Center City to South Philadelphia; costumes inspired by French medieval dress; a "joust" by British officers fighting for the affections of Loyalist women; food and drink; music and dancing; and elaborate flowers and fireworks.

The website losthistory.net says the event became "famous and infamous. 'Famous' because it was staged on a scale that surpassed anything seen in America at the time; 'Infamous' because its critics—rebel, Loyalist, and British alike—were quick to point out that this triumph worthy of Rome was staged to honor a departing general who had won neither a negotiated peace or a military victory."

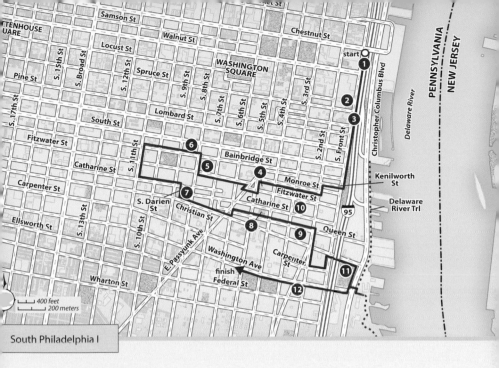

Points of Interest

1. **The Irish Memorial** 100 S. Front St., irishmemorial.org
2. **Philadelphia Korean War Memorial** Penn's Landing
3. **Philadelphia Vietnam Veterans Memorial** Columbus Blvd. and Spruce St.
4. **Meredith Elementary School** 725 S. Fifth St.
5. **Cianfrani Park** Fitzwater and S. Eighth Sts.
6. **The Church of the Crucifixion** 807 Bainbridge St., 215-922-1128, diopa.org/crucifixion
7. **Fiorella** 817 Christian St., 215-305-9222, fiorellaphilly.com
8. **Weccacoe Playground** 400 Catharine St.
9. **St. Philip Neri Church** 220–228 Queen St., 215-468-1922, stphilipneriqueenvillage.org
10. **St. Stanislaus Church** 242 Fitzwater St., 215-468-1922, stphilipneriqueenvillage.org
11. **Gloria Dei (Old Swedes' Episcopal Church)** 916 S. Swanson St., 215-389-1513, old-swedes.org
12. **The Mummers Museum** 1100 S. Second St., 215-336-3050, mummersmuseum.com

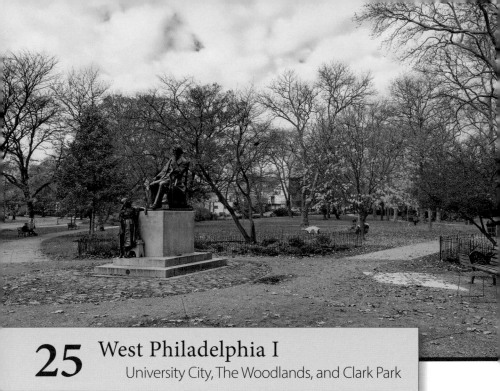

West Philadelphia I
University City, The Woodlands, and Clark Park

Above: West Philadelphia's Clark Park is a popular neighborhood gathering place.

BOUNDARIES: Woodland Ave., Baltimore Ave., 30th St., 44th St.
DISTANCE: 1.6 miles
DIFFICULTY: Easy, with very slight changes in elevation
PARKING: Street parking in this area is very hard to find; a few pay lots serve the hospitals nearby.
PUBLIC TRANSIT: SEPTA bus 30 stops nearby, as does LUCY (Loop through University City), a
shuttle service.

Philadelphia has two rivers. The Delaware, on the east side, serves as the border with New Jersey, while the Dutch-named Schuylkill, pronounced "skool-kul," is the border between Center City and West Philadelphia. The University City area is so called because of its cluster of higher-learning institutions, including the University of Pennsylvania, Drexel University, and the University of the Sciences. This walk introduces the neighborhood, the Woodlands, and Clark Park.

Walk Description

Begin at the University of Pennsylvania's ❶ **Franklin Field,** which has hosted the Penn Relays, the nation's largest track-and-field event, for more than 100 years. The two-tiered stadium, completed in 1925, is the oldest of its kind.

Like Philadelphia, this site has many firsts to its name: the first scoreboard, the first football radio broadcast, the first commercial football game television broadcast, and the first and only place where legendary coach Vince Lombardi's team lost a playoff game. (It was the 1960 NFL Championship Game. The Eagles beat Lombardi's Green Bay Packers 17–13.)

In 1936, Franklin Delano Roosevelt accepted the Democratic presidential nomination here in front of 100,000 supporters. (But note the field was named for Penn founder Benjamin Franklin.) His speech foreshadowed World War II: "To some generations, much is given. Of other generations, much is expected. This generation of Americans has a rendezvous with destiny." Franklin Field was a backdrop for M. Night Shyamalan's 2000 movie *Unbreakable;* the main character was a security guard.

Across South Street is ❷ **The University of Pennsylvania Museum of Archaeology and Anthropology,** aka Penn Museum, founded in 1887. It's one of the world's most renowned archaeology and anthropology research museums and the largest university museum in the country. More than 20 galleries feature a collection of about 1 million items, including a 15-ton Egyptian sphinx and clay tablets covered with Sumerian cuneiform, some of the world's oldest writings. The museum's public gardens feature sculptures by Alexander Stirling Calder and a koi pond.

Continue on South Street. Crossing 33rd Street, the road becomes Spruce Street and heads into the ❸ **University of Pennsylvania's campus.** In the 1700s, the colonies had four colleges—Harvard, William and Mary, Yale, and Princeton—but all catered to the clergy. Benjamin Franklin thought higher education should be open to laypersons, too, stressing practical skills for business and public service as well as the classics. Penn was founded in 1740 and moved here in 1872.

Penn brought the nation these firsts: medical school, business school, and student union organization. Eight signers of the Declaration of Independence and nine signers of the Constitution attended the school.

Continue on Spruce Street, taking in the Collegiate Gothic architecture inspired by England's Oxford and Cambridge universities. At 38th Street, turn left. This is the city's largest collection of food trucks, with fairly priced cuisine in a variety of genres. Visit pennfoodtrucks.com for reviews.

Continue to Baltimore Avenue. Turn right, and bear left to continue on Woodland Avenue. Cross the street to ❹ **The Woodlands,** a historic cemetery home to more than 30,000 people with a Federal-style mansion, a community garden, and an apiary. William Hamilton developed the property in 1786, combining the traditional English garden style with New World plants and practices. Thomas Jefferson called it "the only rival I have known in America to what may be seen in England."

Enter the cemetery, which is still active, and follow the 0.7-mile loop through the grounds. Notables interred here include artist Thomas Eakins and Campbell Soup Company cofounder Joseph Campbell. Bear right after the entrance, and follow the road curving left. Pause at the first intersection. At left, the blackened obelisk topped with an urn marks the graves of a young mother who died during childbirth and her son, who lived less than a year. The engraving reads: "Past the struggle, past the pain/Cease to weep for tears are vain/Calm the tumult of the breast/ They who suffered are at rest."

Continue following the path to the left, passing Hamilton's former home and stables. The Drexel Family Mausoleum is to the right. Family patriarch Francis M. Drexel was an artist and a financial giant whose bank loaned the US government $49 million to finance the Mexican–American War. His son, Anthony, was an adviser to President Ulysses S. Grant and the founder of Drexel University.

Keep on the path. The 90-foot-tall obelisk ahead, the country's tallest funerary monument, marks the graves of Philadelphia dentist Thomas Evans and his family. Evans, who died in 1897, introduced the use of gold to fill cavities, nitrous oxide as an anesthetic, and vulcanite rubber as a base for dentures. While living in Paris, he was dentist to Napoléon III and other members of European royal families. During the American Civil War, Evans advised Napoléon III not to recognize the Confederacy. In his will, Evans designated that part of his fortune establish Penn's dental school.

Continue to exit onto Woodland Avenue. Across the street is the hub for the city's five trolley lines. Known as the Green Lines, the streetcar network is the largest and busiest on the East Coast.

Continue on Woodland Avenue. In 2020, the cemetery partnered with the nonprofit Philadelphia Orchard Project to establish the POP Learning Orchard at The Woodlands. The 1-acre demonstration orchard has 60 fruit and nut trees, pollinator plants, and berry gardens. Crops are donated to local agencies addressing food insecurity.

Turn left on Woodland Avenue, passing through the ❺ **University of the Sciences.** The school, originally called the Philadelphia College of Pharmacy Sciences, was founded in 1821 by local apothecaries seeking to improve standards and professionalize their trade. The university now has four colleges and more than 30 degree-granting programs. William Procter Jr., the father of American pharmacy, was a professor here.

The large black-and-white murals flanking a parking lot before 42nd Street is ❻ *Communion between a Rock and a Hard Place,* a tribute to veterans by veterans. The designs incorporate photos, words, and phrases contributed by a branch of Warrior Writers, a nonprofit that helps veterans articulate their experiences. The organization says the works attempt "to give the viewer the sense of being between two worlds, worlds that are separate, but apart. Veterans can never fully leave either of these two worlds."

Pass Wetherill Way, which is named for the family that has been involved in the university since its start. Four Wetherills were among the college's founders and the legacy of leadership continues: Samuel Wetherill III, a 1968 graduate, served on the university's alumni association and its board of directors. His son, Samuel IV, graduated and serves on the board of trustees.

At 43rd Street, turn right. At right is the main college building with its grand façade.

7 **Clark Park** begins on the left. This 9-acre park, established in 1895 on land donated by banker Clarence Clark, was once an illegal dumping ground. Today it's a hub of community life, with playgrounds, open fields, and multiple picnic options. There's also a Shakespeare in the Park theater company and a large year-round farmers market.

At 43rd Street and Chester Avenue, the fenced garden is the Lower Mill Creek Demonstration Garden and Outdoor Classroom. The University of the Sciences created this open-air classroom in 2001 on land that housed a brick apartment house. It features native plants and showcases best practices in storm water management, including grading the landscape and permeable sidewalks.

Cross Chester Avenue, then cross 43rd Street. In Clark Park, follow the diagonal path on the right. The statue of author Charles Dickens and Little Nell, the tragic heroine of his 1841 novel *The Old Curiosity Shop*, was created for the 1893 Chicago World's Fair. It's one of only three Dickens statues in the world. (Dickens had requested no monument be built in his honor so his writings would stand alone.) Fans gather each February 7 to celebrate Dickens' birthday.

Follow the path to what appears to be an oversize tombstone. This rock, taken from a boulder-strewn hill at Gettysburg Battlefield, is a monument to the doctors and nurses who served at Satterlee General Hospital, the Union's largest army hospital, as well as its 12,700 patients treated. Sisters of Charity nuns nursed the soldiers. In 1903's *West Philadelphia Illustrated,* author M. Lafitte Vieira shared soldiers' memories of one sister, Mother Gonzaga, "whose care of the sick and wounded will remain ever memorable. . . . No matter what the creed, her devotion was ever the same, and not a few soldiers recalled in after years the midnight visits of Mother Gonzaga . . . She was one of the purest and loveliest of women."

Continue on the path to 44th Street and Baltimore Avenue. The walk ends here.

(continued on next page)

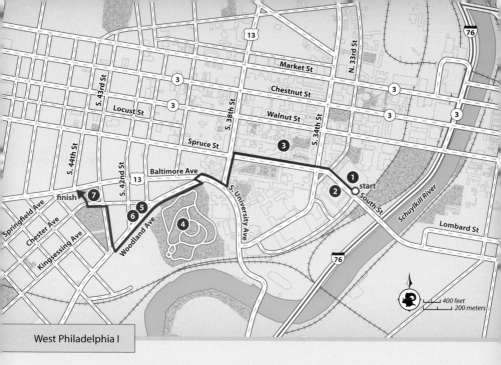

Points of Interest

1 **Franklin Field** 235 S. 33rd St., 215-898-6151, facilities.upenn.edu/maps/locations/franklin-field

2 **The University of Pennsylvania Museum of Archaeology and Anthropology (Penn Museum)**
3260 South St., 215-898 4000, penn.museum

3 **University of Pennsylvania** 215-898-5000, upenn.edu

4 **The Woodlands** 4000 Woodland Ave., 215-386-2181, woodlandsphila.org

5 **University of the Sciences** 600 S. 43rd St., 215-596-8800, usciences.edu

6 **Communion between a Rock and a Hard Place** 4129 Woodland Ave., 989-621-1934,
warriorwriters.org

7 **Clark Park** 4300 Baltimore Ave., 215-568-0830, friendsofclarkpark.org

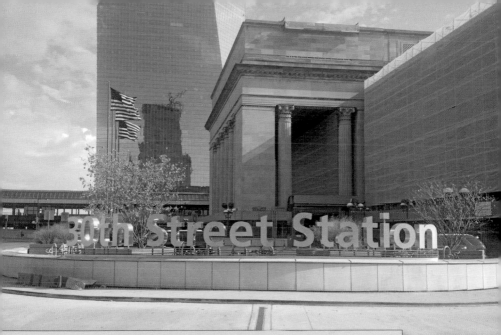

26 West Philadelphia II
30th Street Station, Drexel University, and More

BOUNDARIES: S. 29th St., S. 45th St., Market St., Locust St.
DISTANCE: 3.7 miles
DIFFICULTY: Moderate, with some changes in elevation
PARKING: The tour begins at the train station, which has a pay lot. Street parking can be challenging.
PUBLIC TRANSIT: This tour starts at 30th Street Station, so public transportation is easy. There is a SEPTA subway stop at the station. The following bus lines stop here: 9, 30, 31, 44, 62, 124, 125, and LUCY (Loop through University City).

West Philadelphia is a quick trip from downtown Philadelphia, but early city leaders considered the land on the other side of the Schuylkill River far, far away. In the 1800s, they called it "a great place to put the city's charitable institutions and to remove the pauper class, the insane, and the sickly from Center City," writes author Robert Morris Skaler in *West Philadelphia: University City to 52nd Street*.

Much has changed. West Philadelphia is home to some of the country's best hospitals and universities. Its three-story semi-detached Victorian homes are in high demand. There's a real community spirit too. Notable locals include actor-rapper Will Smith, who proudly sang he was "West Philadelphia born and raised" in *The Fresh Prince of Bel-Air*.

Walk Description

Begin at ❶ **30th Street Station,** which was renamed to honor long-time Congressman and Civil Rights leader William H. Gray III in 2014. Step inside to appreciate the Art Deco–inspired interior's coffered ceilings, chandeliers, and cathedral windows. The building appears in several movies, including *Witness, World War Z,* and *Unbreakable.*

The *Pennsylvania Railroad World War II Memorial* honors the more than 1,300 employees killed in the conflict. It shows archangel Michael lifting a man's body from flames.

Exit via the doors on the opposite side of the station. Turn left. This is The Porch, an outdoor space featuring greenery, seating, and food and beverage trucks. The iron fencing has tree-branch patterns.

Across the street is Drexel Square, the first piece of Schuylkill Yards, a $3.5 billion redevelopment plan led by Drexel University and a private development term. The 1.3-acre square was formerly the parking lot for the *Evening Bulletin,* a daily newspaper in print from 1847 to 1982. The newspaper's office building (3025 Market St.) was also modified, its flat gray wall replaced with a glass-and-brick façade.

Like many cities with universities, Philadelphia has some "Town vs. Gown" tensions. Most recently, the city council took steps to prevent Schuylkill Yards developers from razing an affordable housing development.

Turn left, then pause at Market Street. The former United States Post Office, across the road at 3000 Chestnut Street, was built in the 1930s on land that formerly housed stockyards and slaughterhouses. At the building's dedication, the Postmaster General said it was "second to none in the country." The Postal Service left in 2008 and the IRS moved in.

Rising behind that building is the Cira Centre (2929 Arch St.), a 29-story glass-and-steel structure. Built in 2005, the building's shape appears to change when viewed from different angles. The structure's LED lights change colors and create patterns.

Turn right onto Market Street, with Drexel Square to your right.

Cross S. 31st Street. Look left. Drexel University's ❷ **Paul Peck Alumni Center** was designed by architect Frank Furness to hold the Centennial National Bank during the World's Fair of 1876. Drexel purchased the building in the 1970s and renovated it in 2000.

A few steps farther is a statue of university founder Anthony J. Drexel, a banker and financier who in 1891 spent more than $1.5 million to create the Drexel Institute of Art, Science and Industry.

Walk to 33rd Street. At left is *Mario the Magnificent,* Drexel's dragon mascot. Artist Eric Berg's bronze sculpture, 10 feet high and 14 feet long, is named to honor late alum Mario Mascioli, who didn't miss a basketball game in 25 years.

Continue west. City Square (3401 Market St.) urges its tenants to "Collide Here," and offers examples of what innovations can be the result of these collisions: "Apple might not exist if Steve Jobs and Steve Wozniak didn't live in the same neighborhood. Google might never have been born if Sergey Brin hadn't given Larry Page his tour of Stanford."

Drexel's ❸ **Westphal College of Media Arts & Design** is housed in a Robert Venturi–designed building purchased by the university in 2009 with a $25 million donation from the founder of Urban Outfitters. It became a cutting-edge art center called the URBN Center in 2013. Across the street, the Monell Chemical Senses Center (3500 Market St.) is an independent nonprofit that researches taste and smell. *Face Fragment,* the fiberglass sculpture covered in gold leaf at front, has a pronounced nose and mouth, but the rest of the face appears to have fallen away.

Cross 37th Street to the ❹ **University City Science Center.** Established in 1963, this non-profit is the country's first and largest urban research park, occupying 17 acres. An independent study found that the center's projects past and present annually contribute more than $9 billion to the regional economy.

Cross 38th Street. Look right at 3801 Market Street. *Legacy of Richard Allen* honors the founder of the African Methodist Episcopal Church.

Turn left on 38th Street. The ❺ **Philadelphia Episcopal Cathedral,** built in 1855, is the spiritual home for the 144 congregations of the Episcopal Diocese of Pennsylvania. Its onyx baptismal font was a gift from Anthony Drexel to honor his dead children.

Continue to Chestnut Street and turn left. ❻ **St. Agatha–St. James Roman Catholic Church** was the first Catholic Church west of the Schuylkill River, founded in 1850. In a nod to student schedules, the church offers a 9 p.m. service on Sundays. It offers services in Korean and Spanish.

Neighboring ❼ **Tabernacle United Church,** which hosts both United Church of Christ and Presbyterian congregations, was built in the 1880s. In the 1980s, the church sheltered El Salvadoran refugees. The original sanctuary is now leased to Iron Gate Theater.

Continue on Chestnut Street. ❽ **University Lutheran Church** is called UniLu and has services filled with music, a nod to St. Augustine's remark, "He who sings prays twice." The church welcomes even the most musically challenged: "Hymns play a major part in how we respond to

God's Word. Many members will sing harmony when singing hymns. Others are less musically gifted, but together we always make a joyful noise."

Continue southeast. Cross 36th Street, moving through the Penn campus. This Ivy League university was Ben Franklin's brainchild. Among Penn's distinguished alumni are eight signers of the Declaration of Independence and three US Supreme Court justices. The Electronic Numerical Integrator and Computer, the first all-purpose digital computer, was invented at Penn in 1946, signaling the birth of the Information Age.

Wave Forms (3401 Chestnut St.) features six aluminum bell shapes in a courtyard. The 2007 sculpture evokes "history and modernity, freedom and enclosure, silence and speech. The artist brings forth ideas of dwelling place and the organic, unpredictable nature of change," a university website says.

The grand Georgian Revival building on the corner is Silverman Hall, built in 1900 and part of Penn's law school.

At 34th Street, turn right. Fisher-Bennett Hall (3340 Walnut St.) was originally Bennett College, the first facility built for women on campus, including classrooms, a library, a gymnasium, and a student union. It may be named for Mary Alice Bennett, the first woman to earn a Penn degree. The building now houses the English, Music, and Cinema Studies departments.

Continue on 34th Street. **9** **Fisher Fine Arts Library** is another Frank Furness work. The exterior of the Gothic red sandstone and terra-cotta building, finished in 1891 and restored in the 1990s, features literary inscriptions chosen by Furness's brother, a Shakespearean scholar and Penn faculty member. Melvil Dewey, creator of the Dewey Decimal System, worked with Furness on the interior. Acclaimed architect Frank Lloyd Wright called the building "the work of an artist." It appears in the film *Philadelphia*.

Continue to Spruce Street. Look ahead to see **10** **Penn Medicine,** the University of Pennsylvania's hospital and the Children's Hospital of Philadelphia, the first US hospital dedicated to children's health. The CHOP site was once Philadelphia Almshouse or Old Blockley, a facility "for the poor, the sick, the elderly and the insane—in other words, those individuals who private hospitals have always turned away," the website philaplace.org notes.

Philadelphia boasts many medical firsts—first hospital, first medical school, and first among them. Even today it's estimated that one out of every six doctors in the US trains in Philadelphia.

Turn right onto Spruce Street, passing **11** **Perelman Quadrangle,** a detour-worthy courtyard. The gothic Irvine Auditorium (3401 Spruce St.) was built in the 1930s by architect Horace Trumbauer. Inside is the 11,000-pipe Curtis Organ, one of the world's largest.

Continue on Spruce, walking between buildings that seem suited for Cambridge or Oxford. At 38th Street, lines of food trucks offer cheap but tasty food from around the world. Or stop in the Wawa convenience store (3744 Spruce St.). Wawa is somewhat sacred to locals. Don't mock the name, which comes from the Ojibwa word for a Canada goose. Do not question Wawa: one *Philadelphia* writer wrote a piece about not understanding Wawa's appeal. She received more than 300 dissenting emails.

Cross 38th Street, passing Ryan Veterinary Hospital (3800 Spruce St.), part of Penn's School of Veterinary Medicine.

The University of Pennsylvania Press (3905 Spruce St.) occupies the Carriage House, a 19th-century stable and storage facility belonging to the Potts family. Patriarch Joseph D. Potts was one of the city's wealthiest men. Both of his sons graduated from Penn, then married sisters.

House of Our Own (3920 Spruce St.) is a new and used bookstore in a Victorian house.

Continue to 40th Street. The **12** **Thomas W. Evans Museum and Dental Institute** was appropriately designed with "a frieze of dental tortures," a Penn website notes. Philadelphia native Evans moved to Paris in the 1840s and became the dentist of European royalty, including Napoléon III and his wife, who Evans allegedly helped escape a Parisian mob during the fall of the Second Empire. A display case contains nearly 200 medals, ribbons, and other patient gifts.

Continue on Spruce Street, passing rows of the neighborhood's prized three-story homes. At 42nd Street, look at the church building straight ahead on raised ground before turning right. Penn's Parent Infant Center (4205 Spruce St.) owns this property, but St. Andrew's Chapel, the centerpiece of the now-closed Philadelphia Episcopal Seminary, is sealed but perfectly intact. The wall around the property is Wissahickon schist, a sparkly rock that breaks in straight, flat pieces seen in local structures.

At Walnut Street, turn left. Pass the Restaurant School at Walnut Hill College (4207 Walnut St.).

13 **Masjid Al-Jamia Mosque,** the largest mosque in the city, is housed in a 1920s Spanish Revival–Moorish building that was originally the Commodore Movie Theater. The theater closed in the 1950s. Penn's Muslim Student Association moved into the space in 1973.

Continue west. University City Chinese Christian Church (4501 Walnut St.) and The Association of Islamic Charitable Projects Mosque (4431 Walnut St.) are two examples of creative reuse, as Hidden City Philadelphia notes. The church was a strip mall. The mosque was a Methodist church from the early 1900s.

At South 46th Street, turn right. At Chestnut Street, turn right. Pass West Catholic Preparatory High School (4105 Chestnut St.) to reach the towering **14** **mural of Paul Robeson** on The

Satterlee Apartments. Robeson, who died in 1976, was an actor, athlete, and academic targeted for his civil rights advocacy and Cold War opposition. The New Jersey–born graduate of Columbia University Law School left law to perform in Broadway's *Showboat* and *Othello*. Despite entertaining American troops during World War II, Senator Joseph McCarthy's supporters still labeled him subversive, hurting Robeson's career. Robeson told the House Committee on Un-American Activities, "My father was a slave, and my people died to build this country, and I am going to stay here and have a part of it just like you. And no Fascist-minded people will drive me from it. Is that clear? . . . You are the non-Patriots, and you are the un-Americans, and you ought to be ashamed of yourselves."

Continue east. ⓯ *Building Brotherhood: Engaging Males of Color,* completed in 2015, came from a series of workshops with men of color, ages 12 and older. The workshops asked, "What obstacles get in the way when you seek education and employment?"

Ronald McDonald House (3925 Chestnut St.) occupies the Swain family mansion, built in 1893. In the 1970s, CHOP pediatrician Audrey Evans saw the need for low-cost housing for her patients' families. A fortuitous connection with the Philadelphia Eagles resulted in McDonald's, one of the team's sponsors, funding the first facilities with proceeds from the seasonal Shamrock Shake. Today there are more than 350 facilities worldwide serving ailing children's families.

At South 39th Street, turn left. *Tuskegee Airmen: They Met the Challenge* (16 S. 39th St.) honors the strength and perseverance of the first corps of African American pilots, formed in 1941. The largest image, a pilot's head and goggles, shows the reflection of corps trainer Alfred Anderson. The boy with a model airplane represents the airmen's boyhood dreams.

Continue to Market Street. *The Silent Watcher* (3901 Market St.) is a 19-story mural featuring a female guardian figure watching those around her. It reads, "Maneto Philadelphia: Optimism is a Strategy for Making a Better Future." "Maneto" is Latin for "endure." The quote is from Philadelphia-born Noam Chomsky.

This walk ends here. Cross the Schuylkill River into Center City.

Points of Interest

❶ **30th Street Station** 2955 Market St., 800-USA-RAIL, amtrak.com

❷ **Paul Peck Alumni Center** 3140–3142 Market St., 215-895-2586, drexel.edu/alumni/about/peck

❸ **Drexel University Westphal College of Media Arts & Design** 3501 Market St., 215-895-1834 (visitor center/tours), drexel.edu/westphal

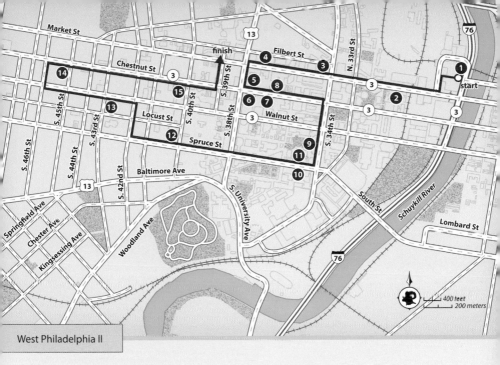

4 The University City Science Center 3711 Market St., 215-966-6000, sciencecenter.org

5 Philadelphia Episcopal Cathedral 23 S. 38th St., 215-386-0234, philadelphiacathedral.org

6 St. Agatha–St. James Roman Catholic Church 3728 Chestnut St., 267-787-5000, saintsaj.org

7 Tabernacle United Church 3700 Chestnut St., 215-386-4100, tabunited.org

8 University Lutheran Church 3637 Chestnut St., 215-387-2885, uniluphila.org

9 University of Pennsylvania Fisher Fine Arts Library 220 S. 34th St., 215-898-8325, library.upenn.edu/finearts

10 Penn Medicine 800-789-7366, pennmedicine.org

11 Perelman Quadrangle 215-898-5552, vpul.upenn.edu/perelmanquad

12 Thomas W. Evans Museum and Dental Institute 4001 Spruce St., dental.upenn.edu

13 Masjid al-Jamia Mosque 4228 Walnut St., 267-275-8087

14 Mural of Paul Robeson 4500 Chestnut St.

15 *Building Brotherhood: Engaging Males of Color* 4008 Chestnut St.

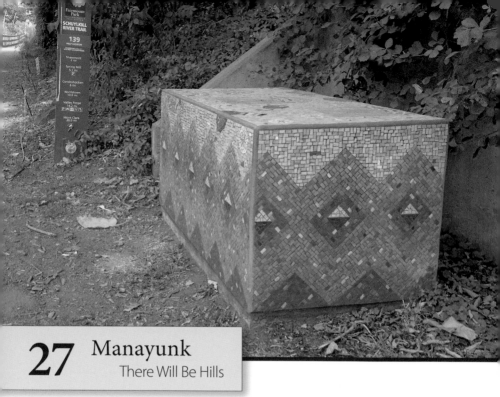

27 Manayunk
There Will Be Hills

Above: A mosaic bench provides a resting place for walkers as they travel along the Manayunk Canal.

BOUNDARIES: Silverwood St., Manayunk Canal Towpath, Lock St., Fountain St.
DISTANCE: 2.5 miles
DIFFICULTY: Moderate, with some changes in elevation and steps
PARKING: Street parking is usually available unless there's a special event.
PUBLIC TRANSIT: The Manayunk SEPTA rail station is at Cresson and Cotton Sts. Bus routes here include the 35 and 61.

Manayunk was once a stand-alone city called Flat Rock. It rebranded itself in 1824, taking its new name from the Lenni Lenape tribe word *manalung*, meaning "river" or "place to drink." That's fitting, as this northwest neighborhood's Main Street is known for its nightlife.

Manayunk was once called the "Manchester of America" because of its thriving factories.

During the 1800s, European immigrants and freed Africans found work in these mills, many of which were devoted to textiles.

Edgar Allan Poe called this part of Philadelphia "one of the real Edens of the land."

Walk Description

Begin at Green Lane and Main Street, under the arches of the massive Manayunk Bridge. This concrete span was built in 1928 by the Pennsylvania Railroad. Southeastern Pennsylvania Transit Authority (SEPTA) used the bridge until 1996. The rails were removed and it opened for pedestrian use in 2015. The Manayunk Bridge Trail now connects Montgomery and Philadelphia counties.

Walk southeast on Main Street. The ❶ **Philadelphia Fire Department's Engine Company 12** was the first city-owned station, built in 1876 when horses carried firefighters to blazes. "The causes of many fires at this time were machinery and locomotive sparks, gas explosions, and arson," writes Thom Nickels, a descendant of one of the neighborhood's oldest families, in *Images of America: Manayunk*. He also notes there was a fierce rivalry between firefighters from Manayunk and those from neighboring Roxborough.

Next door, the Loring Construction Company warehouse fills the former Empress Theater (4441 Main St.). Built in 1914, this former vaudeville and movie palace closed in the 1960s. One local told Hidden City Philadelphia the theater was known as a "scratch theater" when she was growing up because "Movie-goers would come out scratching themselves from flea bites."

Keep an eye out for *Look Long and Look Good,* a series of 30 small murals featuring locals, current and past residents. Most are on Main Street. Artist Mat Tomezsko said half of the featured faces came from archived photos dating to the early 1970s. (Manayunk.com has a scavenger hunt built around the images.)

Continue on Main Street. The ❷ **U.S. Hotel Bar & Grill** has been in operation since 1903. Canal View Park (4430 Main St.) features two mosaics created by artist Josey Stamm and middle school students. Closest to Main Street is *Birds of Fairmount Park,* which contains 83 bird species. The second, *Animals of Fairmount Park,* is on the back of the same building. It appears later in this walk.

Continue on Main, looking left onto Gay Street to appreciate *Under the Rainbow,* an installation of almost 100 multicolored umbrellas suspended 30 feet above the road. It was unveiled in October 2020 to celebrate National Coming Out Day and National LGBTQ+ History Month.

Pass the office of Wm. H. Reichert & Co Printers (4412–16 Main St.), which opened in 1890 but is now only a ghost sign. At Levering Street, turn left. The Levering family were among the first three families to live in Manayunk, with German-born Wigard Levering purchasing 200 acres from William Penn in 1692.

Walk up the incline. **❸** *Sandy's Dream,* on the back of Propper View Apartments, was created with the Sandy Rollman Ovarian Cancer Foundation and is the country's first mural designed to raise cancer awareness. This building formerly housed the Propper Brothers Company, "Manayunk's Busiest Store." In 1911, a woman's summer dress cost less than $2.

At Cresson Street, turn right, walking along a cobblestoned street shaded by the elevated train. This was the area's original commercial district. The El was constructed in the 1930s as a way to prevent train crossing accidents and deaths. Some locals complained the tracks ruined their quaint neighborhood, Nickels writes.

Active businesses operating under the El include **❹ Sorrentino's Deli and Grocery**, known for its Italian hoagie.

Look left and up—and up and up—to see the continuation of Levering Street. This is the **❺ Manayunk Wall,** a sacred, if feared, place in the cycling world. The Philadelphia International Championship is a 124-mile bike race considered the country's most prestigious. The Wall is an 800-meter climb; its steepest section has a 17% grade.

Continue on Cresson Street, passing the *I love Manayunk* mural completed in 2017 by children who signed their "names" in handprints.

At Rector Street, turn left. **❻ St. John the Baptist Roman Catholic Church** is called Manayunk's Cathedral. This Gothic structure dates to the 1890s, when a visiting Irishman donated the equivalent of $1 million to build it. The church organ dates to 1906. St. Katharine Drexel's father was the first organist.

At Silverwood Street, turn left. **❼ St. Josaphat Roman Catholic Church** was founded in 1898. For more than 100 years, these two churches flourished, with each catering to specific immigrant populations. The Irish went to St. John the Baptist, and the Polish went to St. Josaphat. Two other Roman Catholic churches nearby, St. Lucy's and St. Mary of the Assumption, served the Italians and the Germans, respectively.

Continue on Silverwood Street, passing **❽ Pretzel Park,** called Manayunk Park when it opened in 1929. It was renamed, and a silver pretzel sculpture added in 2005, either because its internal sidewalks resemble the twisted treat, or to honor a beloved pretzel vendor. In *Unbreakable,* Bruce Willis's character is seen here with St. Josaphat Church behind him.

Pass Cotton Street, then turn left on Grape Street. Continue to Main Street, cross the road, and turn left.

❾ Pizza Jawn is covered with *The Philly Special,* a mural by artist Jimmy M., who said the colors were inspired by dough and tomato sauce. Jawn is Philly slang. Atlasobscura.com notes that experts say "it's unlike any other word in any other language. It is an all-purpose noun, a stand-in for inanimate objects, abstract concepts, events, places, individual people and groups of people. It is a completely acceptable statement in Philadelphia to ask someone to 'remember to bring that jawn to the jawn.'"

Continue on Main Street, passing the Nickels Building (4323 Main St.), which takes its name from the family of the author of *Images of America: Manayunk*. Built in 1906, it originally housed an F. W. Woolworth store on its first floor and a dance hall above. In the early 1900s, Nickels writes, "dancing was almost as controversial as bootlegging." Christian fundamentalists regularly protested Saturday evening events.

Canal House (4272–4312 Main St.), an upscale apartment building, was once part of Blantyre Mills. It's located at the corner of Cotton Street. Many Manayunk streets are named after the product the closest mill produced, a mill owner, or a prominent local family. During the Civil War, when cotton was hard to come by, this mill began producing woolen blankets for the Union Army.

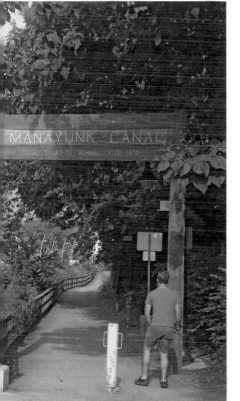

The 2-mile-long Manayunk Towpath was originally used by mules pulling boats along the canal.

When the neighborhood was an industrial hub, Nickels writes, "any adult workers or children could quit or be fired from one mill and within the hour get hired in another." One circa 1860s mill is still in operation. The others have been torn down or converted to residences or commercial spaces.

Canal House and the commercial property across the road at 4313 Main Street are made of Wissahickon Schist, a building stone frequently seen in northwest Philadelphia neighborhoods. The sparkly rock is named for the Wissahickon Creek, where explorers still find small garnets that have fallen out of the stone.

Continue on Main Street. Richards Apex (4202 Main St.) is a fourth-generation family-run metal lubricant company occupying the former Economy Mills, the city's largest textile manufacturer in the mid-1800s.

The ❿ **Manayunk Brewing Company** was a cotton and wool mill in the 1800s. It tapped its first batch of beer in 1996 and now has more than 600 varieties. In 2015, the brewery celebrated Pope Francis's US visit with Papal Pleasure, an ale infused with oak from Malbec wine barrels. A St. John the Baptist priest blessed the brewing water.

Continue, stopping at Shurs Lane to look left. ⓫ **G. J. Littlewood and Son Textile Mill,** the only remaining mill used as a mill, is across the way. Founded in 1869, it's run by the fifth generation of Littlewoods. On the mill's brick wall is *Road Race (Aluminum Bikes),* a collection of brightly colored cyclists made by local business Artesano Ironworks in 2021. Also down Shurs Lane at Cresson Avenue is Rainbow Bridge, a project financed by the Manayunk Development Corporation in 2020 to raise spirits during the COVID-19 pandemic.

Turn around and return to Lock Street. Turn left, then turn right onto the towpath, a 2-mile-long trail mules used while towing boats on the Manayunk Canal. This canal, hand-dug by immigrants in the early 1800s, stretches past Valley Forge, about 15 miles away.

Along the path are multiple sets of steps covered in mosaic. This is *Manayunk Stoops: Heart and Home.* Artist Diane Pieri said neighbors often interact on stoops and the project means "to bring the language of the community to the canal. The stoops are unpretentious yet meaningful reflections of the people and social customs on Manayunk."

Continue on the path, which alternates between gravel, pavement, dirt, and wooden planks. ⓬ **The Venice Island Performing Arts and Recreation Center** across the canal has a theater, sports courts, and a spray garden. The landscaping is designed to handle heavy rains and provides drainage for the entire area: a subterranean stormwater run-off tank can hold almost 4 million gallons of water.

There are opportunities to leave the Towpath at both Rector and Cotton Streets. The paint and mosaic work on the Cotton Street Bridge, by artist Peter Santoleri, is *Tulpenhanink nta,* which means turtle creek in the Native Lenni Lenape language. Santoleri's work appears again later in this walk.

Another possible exit comes at Canal View Park. Look left to see the Philadelphia 76ers mural across the canal, painted in 2021, replacing one that celebrated the area's industrial past. Pass the park steps to see *Animals of Fairmount Park,* a mosaic featuring 50 mammals, reptiles, amphibians, and fish.

Continue, walking under the Manayunk Bridge. Artist Santoleri's *Waters of Change,* a mural blending paint and glass mosaic to depict plant and animal life, begins under the Green Lane Bridge.

Look ahead for a red single-lane bridge, where a gang called the Schuylkill Rangers once ambushed passing boats in the late 1800s. This is Fountain Street. Before the bridge, a slightly uphill path at right branches off from the Towpath. Follow this trail to a business and a white water tower advertising Manayunk Self Storage to exit.

(If desired, continue along the path to see another Santoleri work, *Concrete Tree,* then return to this exit.)

Turn right on Fountain Street to climb the steps covered by *Water Under the Bridge,* a mosaic by Santoleri and Beth Clevenstine. Step back to take in the work as a whole.

At the top, turn right on Umbria Street, passing James Dobson Elementary and Middle School (4667 Umbria St.). Dobson is one of more than 100 buildings designed by Irwin T. Catharine, the school district's architect from 1918 to 1937. In a 2012 article, Hidden City Philadelphia calls Catharine an innovator for his decisions to put gardens and recreation areas on school roofs, add cafeterias to every school so students didn't have to go home for lunch, and replace the outdoor latrine system with boys' and girls' bathrooms on every floor of every school. "As an architect, Catharine has more buildings standing in Philadelphia today than Furness, Trumbauer, Chandler and Kahn combined," with almost all of them being listed on the National Register of Historic Places, the article notes, concluding "it's time to give credit where credit is due and add Irwin T. Catharine's name to the list of Philadelphia's revered architects.

Continue on Umbria to ⓭ **Marchiano's Bakery**, known for its tomato pie and other savory breads. Frank Sinatra was a fan.

Continue to Leverington Avenue and turn right. At Main Street, turn left. *The Liberty Classic* and *The Philadelphia International Championship* by artist Eleanor Dalkner brighten the railroad underpass.

Continue on Main Street with the towpath at right. *Diversity Life in Manayunk* is a community-made mural showcasing local businesses and residents. It is dedicated to Philadelphia Police Officer Garrett Farrell, who was shot and killed in 1980 while chasing a purse snatcher.

Turn left on Green Lane. *Happy Trails* by Alloyius McIllwaine is another mural celebrating biking. The three brightly colored cyclists serve to motivate others on two wheels, the artist told *Manayunk* magazine. Words including "community," "amaze" and "live" also appear in the work. "In a lot of my pieces, I try to include some affirmation," McIllwaine told the magazine. "I like to put a lot of words in my pieces to give it something a bit more tangible."

Continue on Green Lane to the *Welcome to Manayunk* mural. This walk ends here, near where it began.

(continued on next page)

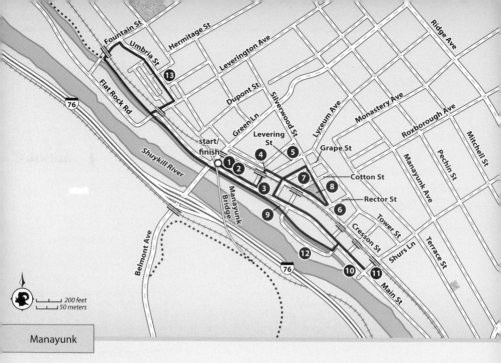

Points of Interest

1. **Philadelphia Fire Department's Engine Company 12** 4447 Main St.

2. **U.S. Hotel Bar & Grill** 4439 Main St., 215-483-9222

3. *Sandy's Dream,* 4368 Cresson Ave., tinyurl.com/sandysdream

4. **Sorrentino's Deli and Grocery** 4361 Cresson St., 215-487-0559

5. **Manayunk Wall** Starting at Levering St. and Cresson St.

6. **St. John the Baptist Roman Catholic Church** 146 Rector St., 215-482-4600, stjohnmanayunk.org

7. **St. Josaphat Roman Catholic Church** 124 Cotton St.

8. **Pretzel Park** 4300 Silverwood St., manayunkcouncil.org/pretzel

9. **Pizza Jawn** 4330 Main St., pizzajawn.com

10. **Manayunk Brewing Company** 4120 Main St., 215-482-8220, manayunkbrewery.com

11. **G. J. Littlewood and Son Textile Mill** 4045 Main St., 215-483-3970, littlewooddyers.com

12. **Venice Island Performing Arts and Recreation Center** 7 Lock St., 215-685-3583, veniceisland.org

13. **Marchiano's Bakery** 4653 Umbria St., 215-483-8585, marchianosbakery.com

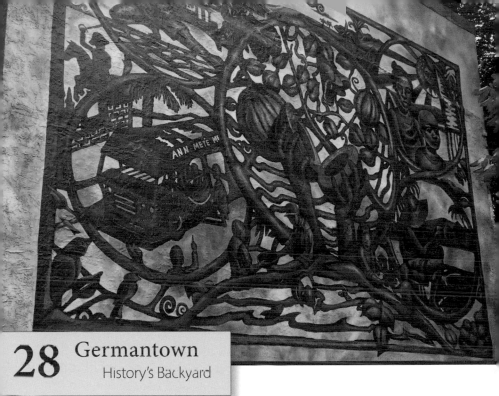

28 Germantown
History's Backyard

Above: Voa Nu, Pwisans Nu (*Our Voice, Our Strength*) *was created by Haitian refugees and locals.*

BOUNDARIES: Abbottsford Ave., Upsala St., Germantown Ave., Greene St.
DISTANCE: 2.8 miles
DIFFICULTY: Moderate, with a few gradual hills
PARKING: This neighborhood is about 30 minutes from Center City Philadelphia. Unless a special event is going on, street parking is easy to find.
PUBLIC TRANSIT: SEPTA's regional train, the Chestnut Hill West, runs from Center City to the Tulpehocken Station. Bus options include the 23 and XH.

It's hard to escape history in Germantown, a neighborhood northwest of Center City. Long before the American Revolution, people with revolutionary ideas—such as ending slavery—settled this rural area known for its rich soil and ample grazing lands.

Germantown, or Germanopolis, was founded by 12 families in 1683 as a separate town a two-hour walk from Philadelphia. Not surprisingly, many of the original residents were from Germany.

Some stops on this tour reference the Revolutionary War's Battle of Germantown, a British victory. For the rebel army, losing this battle a month after Philadelphia had fallen to the British was a huge defeat. About 1,000 colonials were killed or injured, versus about 500 British fighters. Afterward, Washington moved his troops to spend the winter at Valley Forge, from which he launched the sneak attack that changed the course of the war.

Walk Description

Begin at 4650 Germantown Avenue. **❶ Loudoun Mansion,** atop the green hill at left, was built in 1801 on a burial ground, and subsequent generations expanded the structure in different architectural styles. Loudoun is haunted by at least five ghosts, including Little Willie, who died at age 8 in 1860, and the home's last resident, Maria Dickson Logan, who died in 1939. In 1994, Loudoun was severely damaged by fire, but many of the antiques were untouched. It is no longer open to the public.

Walk north on Germantown Avenue. **❷ *Voa Nu, Pwisans Nu (Our Voice, Our Strength)*** was created by members of the city's Haitian community, including some housed in Germantown after Haiti's 2010 earthquake. The work features images important to Haitian culture, including *Le Negre Marron,* an unknown fighter who called on Haitians to fight French invaders.

The former Germantown Settlement Charter School (4811 Germantown Ave.) opened to fanfare in 1999 and closed in scandal in 2010. Its founder reportedly spent millions of taxpayer dollars on the school, only to see its students' test scores drop and its facilities fall apart.

Continue on Germantown Avenue, passing the Fresh Visions Youth Theater (4821 Germantown Ave.). **❸ Hood Cemetery** was founded in 1692 as the Lower Burying Ground. It was renamed in 1850 to honor William Hood, a Philadelphia native who financed the cemetery wall. Hood died in Paris and his body was returned in a barrel filled with brandy. His grave is near the cemetery's entrance. (It's not known if he is still in the barrel.) About 1,000 people are buried here, including soldiers from the Revolutionary War, the War of 1812, and the Civil War.

Continue on Germantown Avenue. The historical marker at 5109 marks where the home of Thones Kunders once stood. (Ancestors say the name is incorrectly spelled on the sign.) Kunders was a cloth dyer who settled here with his family in the 1680s. He hosted the first Quaker Meeting here in 1683, with William Penn in attendance. Four of the congregants wrote the first public document denouncing slavery, 92 years before Pennsylvania was the first state to outlaw the practice.

Continue to Gilbert Stuart Park (5132 Germantown Ave.). Stuart painted portraits of the first six US presidents, including the image of George Washington featured on the dollar bill. Pass Conyngham-Hacker House (5214 Germantown Ave.), which was built in 1775 and is now a multi-family residence.

❹ Grumblethorpe was built in 1744 as a summer home for merchant and wine dealer John Wister. During the Battle of Germantown, British general James Agnew died on the living room floor—the bloodstain is still visible. Agnew's ghost haunts the property. Another ghost reportedly makes herself known by scent, specifically the smell of baking bread.

❺ Trinity Lutheran Church, founded in 1836, was the first neighborhood church offering services in English, not German. The steeple houses the area's first town clock, financed by residents' donations. The church offices occupy the former home of Christopher Sower, who in 1739 printed the colonies' first German-language newspaper. In 1748, he printed the first Bible in Colonial America, a German translation by Martin Luther that predated an English version by 40 years. Despite earning the nickname "The Bread Father" during the Revolutionary War for feeding soldiers' families, Sower was declared a traitor after the conflict for printing a newspaper for British soldiers.

In 1830, author John Fanning Watson wrote the first city history, *Annals of Philadelphia*, in the home at 5275–77 Germantown Avenue. Now online, it provides insights into early city life. The "Punishments" section notes that, in 1735, "Frances Hamilton was punished for picking pockets in the market, by being exposed on the court-house steps, with her hands bound to the rails and her face turned toward the whipping post and pillory for two hours. She was then released and publicly whipped."

Continue to West Coulter Street and turn left. Germantown Friends School (31 W. Coulter St.) opened in 1845 with a class of 33 boys from Quaker families. During the Civil War, students were mocked for their pacifist refusal to fight for either side. In 2002, the school stopped giving academic awards, saying doing so was against Friends' beliefs.

Germantown Friends Meeting House (47 W. Coulter St.) was built in the 1860s, a simple structure in sync with Quaker values.

At Greene Street, turn right. The Pennsylvania School for the Deaf (100 W. School House Ln.) dates to 1820. One of the first headmasters was Laurent Clerc, who taught sign language to Thomas Gallaudet, for whom Gallaudet University is named. This building was used as a hospital during the Battle of Germantown. Six British soldiers are believed to be buried here.

Turn right on West School House Lane. At Germantown Avenue, turn right, walking back toward West Coulter Street. The Deshler-Morris House is also called **❻ Germantown White House** because President George Washington twice used it as a summer retreat. Years before that, British general William Howe claimed the home after his troops defeated Washington's. If the building is open—it has limited hours—step inside to see the Washington family's portrait that includes George, Martha, their grandchildren, and enslaved African William Lee.

Bringhurst House (5448 Germantown Ave.) was the home of carriage-maker John Bringhurst. In 1780, Washington wrote a letter asking an aide to "do me a favour by enquiring & letting me know as soon as possible if any good coachmaker in Phila or GermanTown (Bringhurst for instance) will engage to make me a genteel plain chariot with real harness for four horses to go with two postillions."

At West Coulter Street, cross Germantown Avenue, then turn around. Pass St. Luke's Episcopal Church (5421 Germantown Ave.). Pause at 5425 Germantown Ave. The building that formerly stood here, called Pine Place, was the birthplace of Louisa May Alcott. The *Little Women* author was born on November 29, 1832, her father's 33rd birthday. Alcott's parents were educators who moved to Philadelphia to open a school. The family returned to Boston when Louisa May was 2 years old.

Continue on Germantown Avenue, passing the former home of the Cunningham Piano factory (5427 Germantown Ave.). Founded in 1891, Cunningham is one of the country's most highly respected piano makers and sellers, with customers including Alicia Keys and Usher. When Pope Francis visited Philadelphia in 2016, the company provided the electric organ that accompanied his public Mass.

The small half-acre park in the 5500 block of Germantown Avenue includes the **7** **Historic Germantown Visitor Center,** which has a library with genealogy archives, a neighborhood history museum, and tourist information.

The Impacting Your World Christian Center (5507 Germantown Ave.) is a Victorian building built in the 1880s on the site of a British prisoner-of-war lockup used in the Battle of Germantown. The park's centerpiece is a Civil War memorial featuring a Union soldier standing atop granite from Gettysburg's Devil's Den. The cannon on the north side came from a British ship sunk during the American Revolution.

This area was a hub of 18th-century life with the prison, the stockades, and a marketplace. The website ushistory.org says, "Indian delegations on their way to Philadelphia broke their journeys here."

Continue on Germantown Avenue. *Healing through Faith and Spirituality* (5531 Germantown Ave.) weaves bright patterns and a glass mosaic. Pass through a commercial strip catering to the area's large Muslim population, selling halal meats and women's fashions.

8 **Vernon Park** has a sculpture of John Wister looking oh-so-dapper with his top hat and cane near the entrance. The large Wister clan includes author Owen Wister, whose 1902 novel *The Virginian* romanticized the American West and the cowboy folk hero. The climbing plant wisteria is named for a family member.

During the Civil War, John Wister's iron company supplied ammunition to Union forces. His home, Vernon House, is named either to honor Washington, whose Virginia plantation was called Mount Vernon, or refers to Diana Vernon, a character in Sir Walter Scott's *Rob Roy*.

Continue on Germantown Avenue. The ornate Germantown Town Hall (5928 Germantown Ave.) was city offices but has sat empty since 1998. The interior includes a memorial plaque honoring local soldiers who died in World War I and a bell cast in the same shop as the Liberty Bell.

Pass First United Methodist Church (6001 Germantown Ave.). **9** **Wyck House** was a family residence from the 1750s through the 1970s. Family members include the founders of the Franklin Institute and first horticulture school for women and a designer of the Mexican railway.

At Walnut Lane, turn left. At Greene Street, turn right. **10** **Ebenezer Maxwell Mansion** is a stone Victorian built by the clothing merchant in 1859 for $10,000. The mansion's kitchen includes a line of servants' bells. It's believed this home inspired Charles Addams, creator of *The Addams Family*, who attended the University of Pennsylvania.

At Tulpehocken Street, turn right. Return to Germantown Avenue, then turn right. The marker in the 6100 block of Germantown Avenue recognizes Ora Washington, an African American tennis and basketball phenom who is largely unknown because she was not allowed to compete against better-known white players. She learned the game at the YWCA that once stood here.

Between 1932 and 1942, Washington was the coach and leading scorer of the Philadelphia Tribunes. In a 1988 *New York Times* op-ed, tennis legend Arthur Ashe called the Tribunes "black America's first premier female sports team," noting that white Americans who shunned African American athletics only hurt themselves because "they never got to see Ora Washington of Philadelphia, who may have been the best female athlete ever." During her sporting career, Washington earned money doing domestic work. She died in 1971.

Continue to Herman Street. Cross Germantown Avenue, then turn around to see the **11** **Mennonite Meeting House and Cemetery**, the colonies' first Mennonite church, built in 1708. Before that, Mennonites worshiped with Quakers. This building, made from local stone, replaced the original log structure in 1770.

Continue north. **12** **Johnson House Historic Site** housed four generations of the Johnson family from the 1700s through 1908. During the Battle of Germantown, the pacifist family refused to defend their property, taking refuge in the cellar. The exterior still shows musket ball damage. The Johnsons were also abolitionists, and their home was an Underground Railroad stop. Legend has it that Harriet Tubman and William Still both visited. Its museum began hosting an annual Juneteenth celebration 15 years before the day became a national holiday in 2021.

The 🔞 **Upper Burying Ground** is also called Ax's Burying Ground, after caretaker John Frederick Ax, who maintained the space for 22 years in the 1700s. About 1,300 people are believed to be buried here, but there are only about 300 headstones. Adam Chiseler's headstone notes he died in 1777 at "age 969 years." The one-room Concord School House, built in 1693, sits in one corner. It is either named for the ship that carried the area's first residents from Germany or the phrase "in sweet concord" as people with different religious beliefs lay side by side in the cemetery.

Continue north. 🔞 **Cliveden,** built in the 1760s as Dr. Benjamin Chew's summer home, hosted the Battle of Germantown's bloodiest skirmishes. About 70 soldiers died on Cliveden's grounds. The so-called "Blood Portrait," on the floor of an upstairs bedroom, was allegedly painted by a dying British soldier who used his blood to draw a loved one's face. The image is now faded, but the museum has photos showing the image under a blue light.

A headless woman is said to prowl the grounds. She was allegedly killed by a British soldier who lopped off her head during the fighting and held it aloft to intimidate American soldiers.

Multiple generations of the Chew family owned slaves, and one of the museum's permanent exhibits addresses this history. The mother of Richard Allen, the founder of the African Methodist Episcopal Church, was enslaved here.

This walk of historic Germantown ends here. The Mount Airy tour (page 192) begins about a mile north of here.

Points of Interest

1. **Loudoun Mansion** 4450 Germantown Ave, ushistory.org/germantown
2. *Voa Nu, Pwisans Nu* 4675 Germantown Ave. Mural Arts Philadelphia, 215-685-0750, muralarts.org
3. **Hood Cemetery** 4901 Germantown Ave.
4. **Grumblethorpe** 5267 Germantown Ave., 215-843-4820, philalandmarks.org/grumblethorpe
5. **Trinity Lutheran Church** 5300 Germantown Ave., 215-848-8150

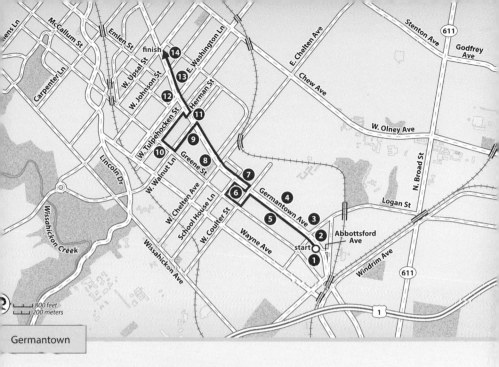

6 **Germantown White House (Deshler-Morris House)** 5442 Germantown Ave., 215-965-2305, nps.gov/inde

7 **Historic Germantown Visitor Center** 5501 Germantown Ave., 215-844-0514, germantownhistory.org

8 **Vernon Park** 5800 Germantown Ave.

9 **Wyck House** 6026 Germantown Ave., 215-848-1690, wyck.org

10 **Ebenezer Maxwell Mansion** 200 W. Tulpehocken St., 215-438-1861, ebenezermaxwellmansion.org

11 **Mennonite Meeting House and Cemetery** 6119 Germantown Ave., 215-843-0943, meetinghouse.info

12 **Johnson House Historic Site** 6306 Germantown Ave., 215-438-1768, johnsonhouse.org

13 **Upper Burying Ground** 6309 Germantown Ave., ushistory.org/germantown

14 **Cliveden** 6401 Germantown Ave., 215-848-1777, cliveden.org

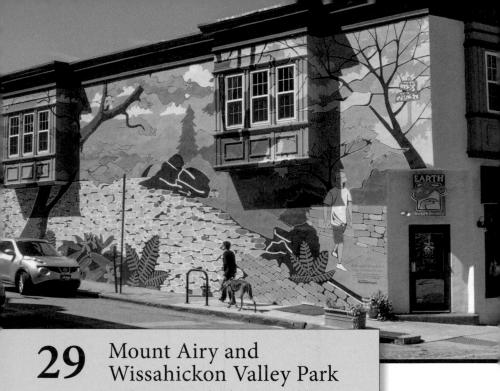

29 Mount Airy and Wissahickon Valley Park

City Meets Suburb Meets Wilderness

Above: Walking the Wissahickon *is a tribute to Mount Airy's natural beauty.*

BOUNDARIES: Germantown Ave., Carpenter Lane, Greene St., McCallum St.
DISTANCE: About 4 miles
DIFFICULTY: Moderate, with some hills
PARKING: There is usually street parking in the area, but note it is zoned for 2 hours only unless you have a residential permit.
PUBLIC TRANSIT: This tour begins and ends at the Allen Lane SEPTA station, making that a great option for transportation. Nearby bus stops include 23 and XH.

Like neighboring Germantown, the Mount Airy neighborhood was founded as a summer getaway and escape from downtown's evils. Europeans began building here in the 1600s. The area takes its name from the home of merchant William Allen, who funded the construction of Independence Hall and Pennsylvania Hospital.

The neighborhood has mansions built for the wealthy, smaller dwellings constructed for laborers, and a modern power station located next to lush Wissahickon Valley Park. CNN's *Money* magazine included Mount Airy in its list of best big-city neighborhoods, along with Brooklyn's Park Slope and Chicago's Lakeview.

Walk Description

Begin at Allen Lane Station (200 W. Allens Ln. at Cresheim Rd.). Built in 1880, the Victorian-inspired regional rail depot has a café and a Little Free Library.

Note the discrepancies between the station and street names. Even locals puzzle over which is correct. SEPTA uses Allen. The city stands by Allens. The Fairmount Park Commission's signs say Allen's. Both station and street are named for William Allen, Chief Justice of colonial Pennsylvania and financier of Independence Hall. Allen's mansion, called Mount Airy, gave the neighborhood its name.

Turn right on Allens Lane. ❶ **Henry H. Houston Elementary School**, a three-story Late Gothic Revival–style building, honors the transportation magnate who ran the Pennsylvania Railroad. Houston oversaw the construction of the 300-home development called Wissahickon Heights and was a trustee for the University of Pennsylvania. Both of his sons attended Penn, and Houston Hall, the country's first student union, is named for the elder son who died in an accident months after his 1878 graduation.

Continue on Allens Lane. The ❷ **Radha Krishna Temple** moved into the former Cresheim Arms Hotel in 1977. About 600 families worship here. Services are open to the public, as is a Sunday vegetarian dinner.

Continue to Germantown Avenue. ❸ **Lutheran Theological Seminary** was founded in 1864 and moved here in 1889. The oldest building on campus, the refectory, dates to the late 1700s. In January 2016, the seminary closed and joined with another to launch the United Lutheran Seminary.

At Germantown Avenue, turn right. The street, once called the Great Road, follows the same path Native Americans used when traveling to points west. The 7200 and 7100 blocks are part of the area's earliest commercial district.

Architect Norman Hulme designed the former Mount Airy National Bank (7208 Germantown Ave.). Hulme also designed English Village for the 1934 World's Fair in New York and helped plan Independence Mall. The neighboring Tourison Building (7200–7206 Germantown Ave.) is an Art Deco gem.

Bioluminescence, on the second floor of 7174 Germantown Avenue, was inspired by the artist's first snorkeling trip in the Caribbean.

Continue on Germantown Avenue. **❹ The Sedgwick Theater,** now the home of the Quintessence Theatre Group, was built in the 1920s during an era of Art Deco movie palaces showing silent films. It closed in 1966. Developers Sedgwick and Ashton Tourison are responsible for the theater and the Tourison building.

❺ Earth Bread + Brewery is an environmentally friendly restaurant. The mural on the building's side, *Walking the Wissahickon,* is a tribute to the beauty of nearby Wissahickon Valley.

The Mount Airy Presbyterian Church complex (13 E. Mount Pleasant Ave.) was built in stages between 1884 and the 1950s. The congregation now worships in the church sanctuary. The rest of the church is being converted to condominiums.

❻ Philadelphia Interfaith Hospitality Network helps homeless families secure permanent shelter. A marketing executive founded the organization after noticing a woman living on the streets near her office. One day, she purchased the woman a sandwich. Soon the executive and her young sons were feeding others. Programming grew from there. *Walking Together*, on the building's side, features the words *service, justice,* and *faith.*

Continue on Germantown Avenue, passing the home fields of Mount Airy Baseball and the Mount Airy peewee football team, The Bantams. (A bantam is a mini version of a regular chicken.)

The **❼ Lovett Memorial Library** opened in 1885 as the Mount Airy Free Library with 421 books in a rented room in a lumberyard, according to the Free Library of Philadelphia. One of the library's supporters, Louisa D. Lovett, was the group's secretary and treasurer, managing its $11.20 budget.

Louisa's aunt, Charlotte Lovett Bostwick, donated land to construct this building. It opened in 1887. By 1891, the library had more than 4,500 books and an annual budget of almost $2,000. The building has since expanded, but some original touches remain, including artwork donated by the Lovett family.

❽ Germantown Home, a nonprofit providing affordable housing and skilled nursing care for seniors, was originally an institution for the very young, according to accessgenealogy.com. In the 1850s, Lutheran reverend William Passavant was visiting the pastor of nearby St. Michael's Church, the Reverend Charles Schaeffer, and his wife, Elizabeth. He wondered if the Lutheran Church could start an orphanage, then gave Elizabeth a dollar, saying, "Now everything must have a beginning: I will give you the first dollar." The Lutheran Orphans Home and Asylum opened in 1859.

The orphanage's population exploded during the Civil War. A list of orphans from 1894 details the children's names and ages; many of the surnames are of German origin, including sisters Catherine and Rosina Breitweiser, ages 10 and 7, and siblings Julius and Pauline Goetz, ages 13 and 11. After a century, the orphanage moved to the suburbs.

Gorgas House (6901 Germantown Ave.) is now office space. The Gorgas family settled in the area in the late 1600s. In 1861, Josiah Gorgas resigned his position in the U.S. Army and moved his family to Virginia to become a major in a Confederacy artillery unit. After the war, he served as headmaster of the College of the South in Sewanee, Tennessee, and president of The University of Alabama in Tuscaloosa.

East Gorgas Lane, at the next corner, is the north border of the Beggarstown community. Its original name was Bettelhausen, a German word with roughly the same meaning and so dubbed because a poor man built the first shack here.

Continue on Germantown Avenue. This area was called Dogtown because, according to William Campbell's *Old Towns and Districts of Philadelphia,* "when it was the custom in Germantown to tie herrings behind bridal coaches, it is said that most of the dogs that followed came from this section." In the 1970s, a local gang co-opted the name. On urbandictionary.com, Dogtown is defined as a "sub-neighborhood in East Mount Airy . . . once a hot-bed of crime . . . that still 'fronts' a hardened appearance." It notes young people wanting to appear tough prefer the name Dogtown to Mount Airy with this example:

> **PERSON #1:** *Dogtown Philly, holla!*
>
> **PERSON #2:** *Whatever, you're from Mount Airy.*

Santander Bank (6740 Germantown Ave.) was built in 1909 for the Pelham Trust Company. In 1911, the bank renovated the basement to create storage vaults for silverware and jewelry "in response to recent robberies in Mount Airy and Germantown," according to Elizabeth Farmer Jarvis's *Mount Airy.*

Continue along Germantown Avenue. Neighboring Trolley Car Park is a grassy square in front of the former trolley depot. The #23 trolley, once a Germantown mainstay, began rattling down the tracks in the 1800s. By the 1920s, this was the country's longest trolley route, beginning north in the Chestnut Hill neighborhood and ending 25 miles later in South Philadelphia. Buses have replaced most trolleys. One old car was part of the now-closed Trolley Car Diner (7619 Germantown Ave.).

Continue to St. Michael's Lutheran Church and Cemetery, active from the early 1700s until the mid-1900s. About 80% of the headstones are unreadable. The earliest legible stone belongs to Mary Elizabeth Hinkle, who died in 1742. As was tradition at the time, bodies were buried with their heads to the east so they would arise facing the sun on Resurrection day. Two can't-miss graves here: The first, to the left of the entrance, honors four Revolutionary War patriots ambushed—"betrayed," the stone notes—by British soldiers. The second, deeper into the cemetery and resembling a table, is the grave of Christopher Ludwig, baker general of the Continental Army. Washington loved his gingerbread. The cemetery is currently closed to the public.

The former Beggarstown School (6669 Germantown Ave.) is a one-room schoolhouse built in 1740.

Cross Germantown Avenue at East Hortter Street, and then turn around. Pass West Phil Ellena Street. In the 1840s, land speculator and druggist George Carpenter built a mansion here and named it Phil-Ellena, meaning "for the love of Ellen," to honor his wife.

Turn left on Westview Avenue, then right on Cresheim Road. Stop at Pelham Road. This residential stretch has homes built in a variety of styles, including Italianate, Georgian, Queen Anne, Norman, Classical, Tudor, Jacobean, and Flemish. "Young architects, who later achieved great distinction, designed these stately homes for newly wealthy Philadelphia businessmen and their families," notes the West Mount Airy Neighbors group.

Turn left on Pelham Road. Pelham was a streetcar suburb within city limits. The Robert M. Hogue home (100 Pelham Road) was designed in the 1890s by the Boyd brothers, among the era's most respected architects, for $20,000.

Continue on Pelham Road. The massive structure at 232 Pelham Road was built in 1897 for William M. P. Braun. It sprawls across 7,600 square feet with six bedrooms and five baths. Note the expansive lawn. Perhaps Braun wasn't worried about trimming it because his father developed lawn-mowing technologies that are still used today.

At Emlen Street, turn right. The Emlen Arms (6723 Emlen St.) is now a public housing complex. Neighboring Pelham Court Apartments (6803–09 Emlen St.) has an open-air entrance that demands a second look. Follow the road as it bears right. **9** **Commodore Barry Club,** also known as the Philadelphia Irish Center, is housed in what was originally the Pelham Auto Club, built in 1905. The Commodore John Barry USN Society purchased the building in 1958. The center promotes Irish culture through music and dance lessons, lectures, and parties. Membership is $25 per year, no Irish heritage required.

Continue to Carpenter Lane and turn left. Pass the Episcopal Church of the Annunciation of the Blessed Virgin Mary (324 Carpenter Ln.) and a home that will remind *Lord of the Rings* fans of Bilbo and Frodo's place in the Shire. Continue on Carpenter Lane, crossing Lincoln Drive. **10** **Big Blue Marble Bookstore** is an independently owned shop and hub of community life. Continue to **11** **Weavers Way Co-Op.** Established in 1973, the co-op moved here in 1974 and now has more than 5,000 household members.

Look across Carpenter Lane at ⑫ **Charles Wolcott Henry School.** Henry, a descendant of a signer of the Declaration of Independence, served on the Fairmount Park Commission, the Philadelphia City Council, and the leadership team of the Young Men's Christian Association of Germantown. When he died in 1903 at age 51, *The Public Ledger* wrote that "the death of a man like Charles W. Henry in the fullness of his activities is a public calamity. He was one of those broadminded and forceful citizens who do not weary nor despair, but keep on doing." Henry's wife, Sallie B. Houston, was the daughter of Henry H. Houston, for whom the first school on this walk was named.

Turn right on Greene Street, walking slightly uphill, then moving downhill after Mount Pleasant Road to reach Carpenter's Woods. "This is a corner of heaven here," poet Gerald Stern wrote, adding he enjoyed lying "for hours with my eyes closed listening to the great sounds." While this walk does not include traversing these woods, it's worth getting lost in its dense, fairy-tale greenery.

Continue on Greene Street. At West Mount Airy Avenue, turn right. Walk to McCallum Street and turn left. (At some points, neighboring bushes almost completely cover the sidewalk.) Make a right at Allens Lane, then a left on Elbow Lane to enter French Village, a collection of Gothic-style homes built by George Woodward. These houses are privately owned today but were rentals in Woodward's time. In *Intimate Bicycle Tours of Philadelphia,* author Patricia Vance describes Woodward as a bit of an eccentric: "He always wore golf knickers and knee socks . . . He used kerosene lamps to read and refused to drive cars with gas engines." The development has some of Woodward's trademarks, including slate sidewalks.

Turn right on McCallum Street. A sign at the driveway across the street says 615/PRIVATE/ CLOSED. Cross the street and walk a few steps down the driveway to reach the public entrance to ⑬ **Wissahickon Valley Park.** Turn right at the trailhead.

Wissahickon Valley has 50 miles of trails. (The Friends of the Wissahickon offers printable trail maps online at fow.org.) Follow the path to the right, walking under the McCallum Street Bridge. Continue to a slight clearing. At left is a bridge over Cresheim Creek. At right is a trail guide. Follow the path to the left of the sign to exit the park.

At the trail's end are the remains of Buttercup Cottage, built in the early 1800s and named after the flowers that filled the grounds. In the late 1800s, two Protestant nuns ran it as a summer rental property for working girls—young women who took seasonal jobs cleaning cottages here. Rent in 1896 was $1/week.

Exit the park on Emlen Street. Turn right and walk up the hill. At Allens Lane, turn left to return to the starting point.

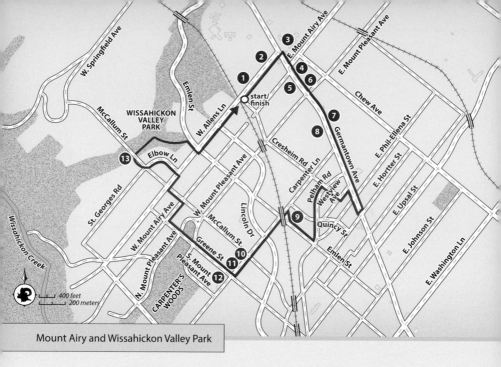

Mount Airy and Wissahickon Valley Park

Points of Interest

1 **Henry H. Houston Elementary School** 135 W. Allens Lane

2 **Radha Krishna Temple** 41 W. Allens Lane, 215-247-4825, iskconphiladelphia.com

3 **Lutheran Theological Seminary of Philadelphia (now the United Lutheran Seminary)** 7301 Germantown Ave., 215-248-4616, unitedlutheranseminary.edu

4 **Quintessence Theatre Group (formerly The Sedgwick Theater)** 7137 Germantown Ave., 215-987-4450, quintessencetheatre.org

5 **Earth Bread + Brewery** 7136 Germantown Ave., 215-242-6666, earthbreadbrewery.com

6 **Philadelphia Interfaith Hospitality Network** 7047 Germantown Ave., 215-247-4663, philashelter.org

7 **Lovett Memorial Library** 6945 Germantown Ave. For more information, contact the Free Library of Philadelphia: 215-686-5322, freelibrary.org.

8 **Germantown Home** 6950 Germantown Ave., 215-848-3306, germantownhome.org

9 **Commodore Barry Club (Philadelphia Irish Center)** 6815 Emlen St., 215-843-8051, theirishcenter.com

10 **Big Blue Marble Bookstore** 551 Carpenter Lane, 215-844-1870, bigbluemarblebooks.com

11 **Weavers Way Co-op** 559 Carpenter Lane, 215-843-2350, weaversway.coop

12 **Charles Wolcott Henry School** 601–645 Carpenter Lane

13 **Wissahickon Valley Park** McCallum Street between West Mermaid Lane and West Allens Lane, 215-247-0417, fow.org

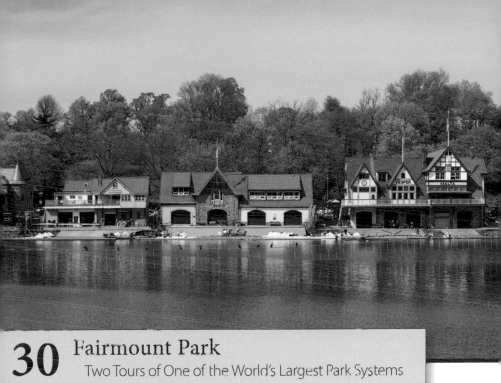

30 Fairmount Park
Two Tours of One of the World's Largest Park Systems

East Fairmount Park

BOUNDARIES: Waterworks Dr., Mount Pleasant Dr., Schuylkill River, N. 33rd St.
DISTANCE: 3.8 miles
DIFFICULTY: Moderate, with some changes in altitude
PARKING: Street parking is available on side roads.
PUBLIC TRANSIT: SEPTA bus routes include the 25, 43, 89, and MFL.

Fairmount Park is the overarching name for the city's park system, composed of 63 parks and more than 9,000 acres of greenery. This walk focuses on one 2,050-acre section that most Philadelphians consider the "real" Fairmount Park.

In 2016, website SquareFoot compared the size of this small stretch of park with Manhattan's often-vaunted Central Park. The results were embarrassing—for New York, that is. Fairmount Park tops 4,000 acres, making it almost five times as large as Central Park, which covers 843 acres.

There are many park guides available. The first tour explores the park's eastern segment; the second, the western part. While the distances covered are longer than other tours, the write-ups are actually shorter, as some stretches simply feature nature.

The end of the East Fairmount Park walk is close to the start of the West Fairmount Park tour.

Walk Description

Begin at ❶ **Fairmount Water Works,** the nation's first municipal water-treatment center, tucked behind the Philadelphia Museum of Art. The water part of this complex, made up of a dam, pump house, and reservoir, was built between 1819 and 1822 to ensure clean drinking water. The accompanying buildings—including the superintendent's house and the pavilions—are considered some of the city's loveliest architecture. The whole project was a tourist draw in the 1800s. Only Niagara Falls drew more visitors.

The Fairmount Water Works Interpretive Center allows visitors to create a rainstorm and follow the water as it drains. Wander and enjoy the fabulous view. Edgar Allan Poe's ghost reportedly walks near the water at night. (Poe's ghost has also been spotted at the Spring Garden home where he wrote part of "The Raven.")

Exit by walking toward Kelly Drive. Near the road is the Garden of Heroes, which honors Europeans who "threw themselves into the cause of emancipating the colonies from the yoke of British tyranny," including the Marquis de Lafayette of France, Poland's General Casimir Pulaski, General Friedrich von Steuben of Prussia, and British General Richard Montgomery.

Turn left on Kelly Drive. The boating clubs of ❷ **Boathouse Row** are members of the Schuylkill Navy, the oldest amateur athletic governing body in the country and host of major rowing competitions, including the Aberdeen Dad Vail Regatta, the Head of the Schuylkill, and the Stotesbury Cup Regatta. Many Olympic athletes have trained on the river, including John B. Kelly Jr., a four-time Olympian who brought home a bronze medal after the 1956 games in Australia. Kelly was the brother of actress Grace Kelly. Their father, John B. Kelly Sr., was also an accomplished rower, winning three gold medals in two Olympic Games. While Kelly Drive is named for Kelly Jr., a statue of Kelly Sr. is along the river near the viewing stands.

Follow the path along the river. The sculpture *Thorfinn Karlsefni* remembers a Viking believed to have come to America in 1004. *Stone Age in America* depicts a native woman protecting her child from attack. When the trail splits, follow either path, as they reconnect later.

The plaza-type area with statues is the central terrace of the Ellen Phillips Samuel Memorial sculpture garden. The bronze work at center is *The Spirit of Enterprise*.

Continue, passing Brewery Hill Drive. *Playing Angels* features three winged figures dancing to unheard music.

This walk leaves the river on Fountain Green Drive. To see the statue of John B. Kelly Sr. and the race-viewing stands, continue for about 0.5 mile, then double back.

On Fountain Green Drive, a sign marks THE BOXERS' TRAIL. Forget Rocky; this path has been used by real boxers past and present for training. Muhammad Ali came here looking for Joe Frazier before their famous bout.

Continue to Mount Pleasant Drive. Turn left, following the road to ❸ **Mount Pleasant Mansion,** an 18th-century Georgian home built by Captain John Macpherson, a privateer. John Adams once said Macpherson had "an arm twice shot off." Benedict Arnold also owned this house, but he fled the country before he could move in.

Mount Pleasant Mansion is one of six "Charms," historic homes from the 1700s built as summer houses for the wealthy.

Continue on Mount Pleasant Drive until it ends. Turn right onto Reservoir Drive. Bear left as the road winds, then make a definitive right on an extension of Reservoir Drive to visit ❹ **Smith Memorial Playground and Playhouse.** The 16,000 square-foot play mansion features a 44-foot wooden slide, a giant seesaw, and other delights for the 10-and-under crowd.

The Richard and Sarah Smith Trust created this 6.5-acre play area in the late 1880s to honor their son, Stansfield, who died at age 40. The Smiths made their fortune in the typesetting business.

Leave Smith Playground, returning to Reservoir Drive. Turn right. ❺ **Sedgley Woods Historic Disc Golf Course** is free to the public; BYOF (Bring Your Own Frisbee).

Walk to North 33rd Street and turn right. The 33rd Street Bridge is covered with black-and-white scenes paying homage to the surrounding neighborhoods, including Brewerytown and Strawberry Mansion. Look for John Coltrane, the late jazz great who lived nearby.

Continue to Girard Avenue. Turn left to return downtown. Turn right to pick up the West Fairmount Park walk, which begins at nearby Lansdowne Drive.

West Fairmount Park

BOUNDARIES: Girard Ave., Montgomery Dr., Lansdowne Dr., States Dr.
DISTANCE: 3.9 miles
DIFFICULTY: Moderate, with some changes in elevation

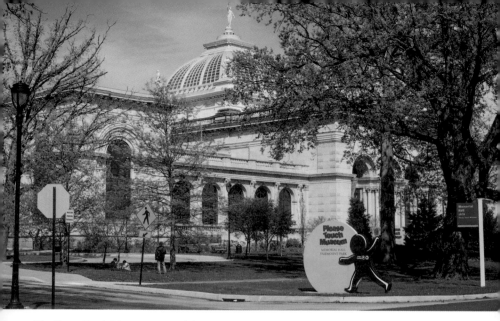

The Please Touch Museum is one of the country's finest children's museums. It's housed in a building that was constructed for the 1876 centennial celebration.

PARKING: There are multiple pay lots near the zoo.
PUBLIC TRANSIT: SEPTA bus routes include the 5, 15, 15B, and MFL.

In 1876, Philadelphia celebrated the nation's 100th birthday by hosting the country's first World's Fair, also called the Centennial International Exposition. More than 10 million people visited during the six-month event. The most notable remaining structure is the Please Touch Children's Museum.

Walk Description

Start at ❶ **The Philadelphia Zoo.** The nation's first zoo was established by charter in 1859, but the Civil War postponed its opening for 15 years. Adult admission was 25 cents; children's tickets were 10 cents. Those prices held for 50 years. The original zoo had its own wharf for visitors arriving by steamboat.

Today, the 42-acre property is home to more than 1,300 animals, including Betsy and Benjamin, two red pandas born in 2015. The zoo averages more than 1 million visitors annually. Inside the main gates is The Solitude, a home designed and built by William Penn's grandson. George Washington once dined here.

From the zoo entrance, cross North 34th Street, and turn left on North 34th Street (which turns into Lansdowne Drive), taking the sidewalk under the bridge decorated with giraffe neck mosaics. The School of the Future (4021 Parkside Ave.) is a public high school designed in partnership with Microsoft. Ahead, Lansdowne Drive splits. Turn right.

At the traffic circle, take the second right to reach the Smith Civil War Memorial Arch. Completed in 1912, the structure honors Civil War generals, including McClellan and Meade. It was financed by Sarah and Richard Smith, who also endowed Smith Playground. There's a tiny statue of Smith, in his typesetter's apron, high on the memorial.

Pass through the arch, now on Avenue of the Republic. The ❷ **Please Touch Museum** is housed in Memorial Hall, once part of the Centennial Exposition. The structure was built without wood to be fireproof and cost $1.5 million to complete, an incredible amount for 1876. The museum has 25,000 toys. Popular exhibits include Alice in Wonderland and the grocery store. The piano from the movie *Big* is here, and young guests can jump on the keys. Built in the early 1900s, the Woodside Park Dentzel Carousel features more than 50 hand-carved animals, with a few cats, pigs, goats, and rabbits among the horses.

Continue straight and cross Belmont Avenue. At Avenue of the Republic's end is the ❸ **Catholic Total Abstinence Union Fountain.** Commissioned for the Centennial Exposition, the fountain has Moses at center holding the Ten Commandments. Medallions around the base represent high-profile Catholics from the Revolutionary War, including the Marquis de Lafayette. All four larger-than-life statues outside the basin originally had working water fountains.

Continue to ❹ **Mann Center for the Performing Arts,** which opened in 1935 as a summer performing space for the Philadelphia Orchestra called Robin Hood Dell Concerts. Renamed to honor businessman and supporter Frederic R. Mann, the venue now welcomes all performers.

Exit the circle via States Drive, the unmarked road to the right. Continue to Belmont Avenue. The Ohio House (4700 States Dr.), on the left, is the other park building from the Centennial Exhibition.

Turn left on Belmont Avenue, then right on Montgomery Drive. At Belmont Mansion Drive, turn right, which becomes Horticultural Drive. The ❺ **Fairmount Park Horticulture Center** includes an arboretum, a demonstration garden, a vegetable garden, a reflecting pool, a pavilion, and a butterfly garden. Picnicking is allowed with a permit. The center's sundial is the work of sculptor Alexander Stirling Calder, whose father created the William Penn statue atop City Hall.

Follow the road to the left to see *The Journeyer,* a statue commissioned for the bicentennial celebration.

Continue to ❻ **Shofuso Japanese House and Garden.** Originally displayed on the grounds of New York's Museum of Modern Art, this small building is a reconstruction of a 17th-century scholar's home and teahouse. The garden has a pool and cherry blossom trees. Shofuso hosts an annual Cherry Blossom Festival, as its collection of trees rivals Washington, D.C.'s.

Shofuso also features tea ceremonies performed by members of the Kyoto-based Urasenke tea school. This 450-year-old practice is an art form. (Advance registration is advised.) Other programming includes lessons in Japanese flower-arranging and mask-making workshops.

Turn left on Lansdowne Drive, passing the rear of the Please Touch Museum. At the T intersection, turn left. Continue on Lansdowne Drive to end your walk at the Philadelphia Zoo.

Points of Interest

East Fairmount Park

1. **Fairmount Water Works** 640 Waterworks Dr., 215-685-0723, fairmountwaterworks.org
2. **Boathouse Row** 1 Boathouse Row, 215-685-3936, boathouserow.org
3. **Mount Pleasant Mansion** Mount Pleasant Drive, 215-763-8100, parkcharms.org
4. **Smith Memorial Playground and Playhouse** 3500 Reservoir Drive, 215-765-4325, smithplayground.org
5. **Sedgley Woods Historic Disc Golf Course** N. 33rd and Oxford Sts., sedgleywoods.com

The Philadelphia Zoo, the nation's first, averages more than 1 million visitors each year.

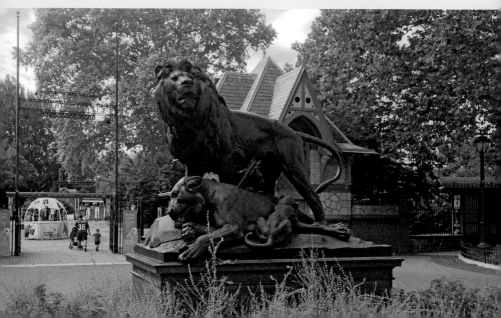

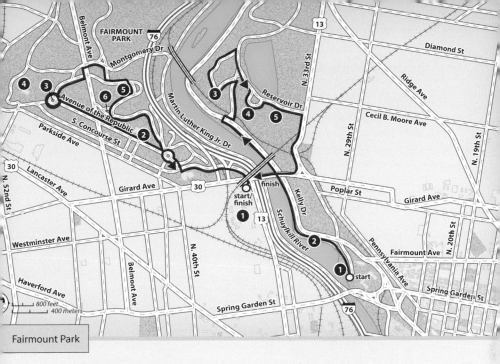

West Fairmount Park

1. **The Philadelphia Zoo** 3400 W. Girard Ave., 215-243-1100, philadelphiazoo.org

2. **Please Touch Museum** 4231 Avenue of the Republic, 215-581-3181, pleasetouchmuseum.org

3. **Catholic Total Abstinence Union Fountain** Avenue of the Republic and States Street

4. **Mann Center for the Performing Arts** 5201 Parkside Ave., 215-546-7900, manncenter.org

5. **Fairmount Park Horticulture Center** 100 North Horticultural Drive, 215-685-0096, phila.gov

6. **Shofuso Japanese House and Garden** Lansdowne and Horticultural Drives, 215-878-5097, japanphilly.org/shofuso

Appendix I: Walks by Theme

Architectural Tours

Arts and Culture

Family Fun

Independence National Park (Walk 1)

The Museum District: From Love Park to the *Rocky* Steps (Walk 4)

Fitler Square and the Schuylkill River (Walk 7)

South Broad Street II: From the Avenue of the Arts to
    Franklin Delano Roosevelt Park (Walk 11)

Market Street East: The Gayborhood and Reading Terminal Market (Walk 12)

Along the Delaware River (Walk 15)

Old City (Walk 16)

Northern Liberties (Walk 18)

The River Wards: Kensington and Fishtown (Walk 19)

Fairmount, the Neighborhood (Walk 20)

South Philadelphia I (Walk 23)

West Philadelphia I: University City, The Woodlands, and Clark Park (Walk 25)

Manayunk (Walk 27)

Mount Airy and Wissahickon Valley Park (Walk 29)

Fairmount Park (Walk 30)

Green Spaces

The Museum District: From Love Park to the *Rocky* Steps (Walk 4)

The Museum District: From the Art Museum to the Cathedral (Walk 5)

Rittenhouse Square (Walk 6)

Fitler Square and the Schuylkill River (Walk 7)

South Broad Street II: From the Avenue of the Arts to
    Franklin Delano Roosevelt Park (Walk 11)

Along the Delaware River (Walk 15)

Old City (Walk 16)

South Philadelphia II (Walk 24)

West Philadelphia I: University City, The Woodlands, and Clark Park (Walk 25)

Manayunk (Walk 27)

Germantown (Walk 28)

Mount Airy and Wissahickon Valley Park (Walk 29)

Fairmount Park (Walk 30)

History

Independence National Park (Walk 1)

African American Philadelphia (Walk 3)

South Broad Street II: From the Avenue of the Arts to Franklin Delano Roosevelt Park (Walk 11)

History *(continued)*

Market Street East: The Gayborhood and Reading Terminal Market (Walk 12)
Old City (Walk 16)
Society Hill (Walk 17)
Antiques Row, Jewelers' Row, and Rittenhouse Row (Walk 21)
Headhouse Square, Fabric Row, and South Street (Walk 22)
Germantown (Walk 28)

Appendix II: Sources of Information

Websites

Association for Public Art associationforpublicart.org

Atlas Obscura atlasobscura.com

Billy Penn billypenn.com

Center City District centercityphila.org

City of Philadelphia phila.gov

Constitutional Walking Tour of Philadelphia theconstitutional.com

Curbed Philly philly.curbed.com

The Delaware River Blog delawareriver.net

Delaware River Waterfront Corporation delawareriverwaterfront.com

Discover Philadelphia discoverphl.com

Eater Philly philly.eater.com

The Encyclopedia of Greater Philadelphia philadelphiaencyclopedia.org

Explore Pennsylvania History, part of the Commonwealth's
Department of Community and Economic Development explorepahistory.com

Fairmount Park Conservancy myphillypark.org

Free Library of Philadelphia freephilly.org

Friends of Wissahickon fow.org

Ghost Sign Project ghostsignproject.com

Greater Philadelphia Cultural Alliance philaculture.org

Hidden City Philadelphia hiddencityphila.org

Historic Houses of Fairmount Park parkcharms.com

Historic Philadelphia historicphiladelphia.org

The Historical Marker Database hmdb.org

Historical Society of Philadelphia hsp.org

Independence Hall Association ushistory.org

Independence Visitor Center phlvisitorcenter.com

Kenneth W. Milano kennethwmilano.com

Mural Arts Philadelphia muralarts.org

Naked Philly ocfrealty.com/naked-philly

Newspapers.com

Pennsylvania Academy of Fine Arts pafa.org

Pennsylvania Heritage paheritage.com

Pennsylvania Historical and Museum Commission phmc.pa.gov

Philadelphia phillymag.com

Philadelphia Business News bizjournals.com/philadelphia

Philadelphia Church Project phillychurchproject.com

Philadelphia Citizen thephiladelphiacitizen.org

Philadelphia Convention and Visitors Bureau discoverphl.com

The Philadelphia Gayborhood Guru thegayborhood.guru.wordpress.com

Philadelphia History Museum philadelphiahistory.org

The Philadelphia Inquirer, The Philadelphia Daily News, and Philly.com philly.com

Philadelphia Public Art philart.net

Philadelphia's Magic Gardens phillymagicgardens.org

PhilaPlace philaplace.org

Philebrity philebrity.com

Philly History Blog phillyhistory.org/blog

PhillyMuralPics.com phillymuralpics.com

Phillyvoice phillyvoice.com

PlanPhilly planphilly.com

Smithsonian smithsonian.org

South Street Headhouse District southstreet.com

Southwark Historical Society southwarkhistory.org

Spirit News spiritnews.org

Streets Dept streetsdept.com

US National Park Service nps.gov

Visit Philadelphia visitphilly.org

Wee Wander wee-wander.com

WHYY whyy.org

Wooder Ice wooderice.com

Workshop of the World Philadelphia workshopoftheworld.com

YIMBY phillyyimby.com

Print Sources

Avery, Ron. *City of Brotherly Mayhem: Philadelphia Crimes & Criminals.* Philadelphia: Otis Books, 1997.

Baker, Irene Levy. *100 Things to Do in Philadelphia Before You Die.* St. Louis: Reedy Press, 2020.

Booker, Janice L. *Philly Firsts: The Famous, Infamous, and Quirky of the City of Brotherly Love.* Philadelphia: Camino Books, 1999.

Brenner, Roslyn. *Philadelphia's Outdoor Art.* Philadelphia: Camino Books, 2002.

Brown, Dotty. *Boathouse Row: Waves of Change in the Birthplace of American Rowing.* Philadelphia: Temple University Press, 2016.

Cooper, George. *Poison Widows: A True Story of Witchcraft, Arsenic, and Murder.* New York: Thomas Dunne Books, 1999.

Dubin, Murray. *South Philadelphia: Mummers, Memories, and the Melrose Diner.* Philadelphia: Temple University Press, 1996.

Flanagan, Jeffrey Michael. *On the Backs of Horses: The Great Epizootic of 1872.* UK: CORE, 2011.

Gallery, John Andrew. *Philadelphia Architecture: A Guide to the City.* Philadelphia: Paul Dry Books, 2016.

Golden, Jane, Robin Rice and Natalie Pompilio. *More Philadelphia Murals and the Stories They Tell.* Philadelphia: Temple University Press, 2006.

Graham, Kristen A. *A History of the Pennsylvania Hospital.* Charleston, SC: The History Press, 2008.

Jarvis, Elizabeth Farmer. *Images of America: Mount Airy.* Charleston, SC: Arcadia Publishing, 2008.

Kyriakodis, Harry. *Northern Liberties: The Story of a Philadelphia River Ward.* Charleston, SC: The History Press, 2012.

Litchman, Lori. *A Philadelphia Story: Founders and Famous Families from the City of Brotherly Love.* Covington, KY: Clerisy Press, 2016.

Milano, Kenneth W. *Remembering Kensington & Fishtown: Philadelphia's Riverward Neighborhoods.* Charleston, SC: The History Press, 2008.

Murphy, Jim. *Real Philly History, Real Fast.* Philadelphia: Temple University Press, 2021.

Nickels, Thom. *Images of America: Manayunk.* Charleston, SC: Arcadia Publishing, 2001.

Northern Liberties Neighbors Association. *Guide to Northern Liberties.* Philadelphia: Northern Liberties Neighbors Association, 1982.

O'Toole, Lawrence. *Fading Ads of Philadelphia.* Charleston, SC: The History Press, 2012.

Pompilio, Natalie and Tricia. *This Used To Be Philadelphia.* St. Louis: Reedy Press, 2021.

Ristine, James D. *Philadelphia's Fairmount Park.* Charleston, SC: Arcadia Publishing, 2005.

Saffron, Ina. *Becoming Philadelphia: How an Old American City Made Itself New Again.* New Brunswick, NJ: Rutgers University Press, 2020.

Skaler, Robert Morris. *Images of America: Philadelphia's Broad Street, South and North.* Charleston, SC: Arcadia Publishing, 2003.

Skaler, Robert Morris and Thomas H. Keels. *Images of America: Philadelphia's Rittenhouse Square.* Charleston, SC: Arcadia Publishing, 2008.

Skaler, Robert Morris. *Images of America: Society Hill and Old City.* Charleston, SC: Arcadia Publishing, 2005.

Skaler, Robert Morris. *Images of America: West Philadelphia, University City to 52nd Street.* Charleston, SC: Arcadia Publishing, 2002.

Smith, Irina and Ann Hazan. *The Original Philadelphia Neighborhood Cookbook.* Philadelphia: Camino Books, 1988.

Vance, Patricia. *Intimate Bicycle Tours of Philadelphia.* Philadelphia: University of Pennsylvania Press, 2004.

Wurman, Richard Saul and John Andrew Gallery. *Man-Made Philadelphia: A Guide to Its Physical and Cultural Environment.* Cambridge, MA: The MIT Press, 1972.

Index

About the Author

Freelance journalist **Natalie Pompilio** lives in an alley off an alley in South Philadelphia. A former staff writer with *The Times-Picayune* (New Orleans), *The Philadelphia Inquirer,* and *The Philadelphia Daily News,* she is a frequent contributor to *The Star-Ledger* (Newark), *The Washington Post,* the *Associated Press,* and regional magazines. She and her sister also collaborated on *This Used to Be Philadelphia* (Reedy Press, 2021). Her other books include *More Philadelphia Murals and The Stories They Tell* (with Jane Golden and Robin Rice, Temple University Press, 2006) and *Philadelphia A to Z* (with photographer Jennifer Zdon, self-published, 2009).

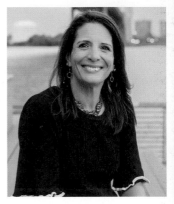

photo credit: Tricia Pompilio

Natalie's idea of a perfect night is sitting on her roof deck on a warm night with her husband, Jordan Barnett, and watching the chimney swifts do their nightly dance. Read more of her work at nataliepompilio.com.

About the Photographer

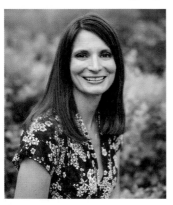

Tricia Pompilio is a Philadelphia-based portrait and family photographer. Her favorite subjects are dancers and families, especially her husband, Vince Savarese, and their three daughters, Fiona, Luna, and Poppy. In 2019, *Philadelphia Family* magazine named her the city's best portrait photographer. When she's not behind the camera, she's probably rereading Harry Potter while listening to Rob Thomas while her cats, Albus and Clara, sleep at her feet. Follow her work at triciapompiliophotography.com and on Instagram at triciapphotography.

photo credit: Karen Schanely Photography